Sub-clinical
Lead Poisoning

Sub-clinical Lead Poisoning

H. A. WALDRON
Department of Social Medicine
The Medical School,
Birmingham, England

D. STÖFEN
Montabaur
West Germany

P 134–142
156

ACADEMIC PRESS 1974 LONDON NEW YORK
A Subsidiary of Harcourt Brace Jovanovich, Publishers

ACADEMIC PRESS INC. (LONDON) LTD
24–28 Oval Road,
London NW1

U.S. Edition published by
ACADEMIC PRESS INC.
111 Fifth Avenue,
New York, New York 10003

Library of Congress Catalog Card Number: 73–19022
ISBN: 0–12–671650–1

Text set in 11/12 pt. Monotype Baskerville, printed by letterpress,
in Great Britain at The Pitman Press, Bath

Preface

As a clinical entity lead poisoning has become rare. The number of deaths attributable to this cause has fallen to a very low figure during the course of this century and the number of cases of industrial poisoning shows a similar decline. Nevertheless, the use of lead is increasing particularly for the manufacture of lead alkyls for antiknock agents in petrol and there has been much speculation in recent years as to whether the massive release of lead into the environment consequent upon its use in petrol is having an adverse effect on the health of the general population. Much of the argument which has ensued has been heated and there has been a tendency for extremists on both sides to take refuge behind their firmly entrenched positions.

In this book we have tried to assess the information available to us from all sources, including eastern Europe where the problem of sub-clinical lead poisoning has been considered for longer than in the west, and present the evidence in such a way that reasonable and reasoned conclusions may be drawn from it.

To put sub-clinical effects into perspective we have included an account of the metabolism and pathological effects of lead and of the signs and symptoms of clinical poisoning. We hope these chapters will be of use not only to those who are interested in environmental aspects of lead but also to those whose main concern is for clinical poisoning.

The bibliography of lead poisoning is of daunting dimensions and whilst we have tried to include what we see as the most significant contributions we are well aware that there will be many who feel that not only have we made serious errors of inclusion and omission but that many up-to-date pieces of work are absent. To those who think that these faults seriously affect the arguments presented here we offer our apologies and hope that there may be an opportunity to redress the balance in the future.

Acknowledgements

This book owes much to the help and encouragement given to the authors by friends and colleagues. We would like to thank particularly Dr W. Becker, Professor Th. Bersin, Dr H. Harmsen, Dr H. R. Kanitz, Dr A. C. Rubis, Dr A. Schatz and Dr P. G. Seeger. During its various stages of preparation the manuscript was read by Professor D. Bryce-Smith, Dr R. Stephens and Dr G. Stratford, each of whom corrected errors of fact, style and grammar, in addition to pointing out those passages which were unclear or poorly argued. Such merits as the book may have are largely due to their efforts, whilst the defects remain the sole responsibility of the authors.

A number of the illustrations are from original photographs which were given to us for inclusion by Dr R. Astley of the Birmingham Children's Hospital (Fig. 49), Professor B. Clayton of the Hospital for Sick Children, Great Ormond Street (Fig. 50), Professor L. S. Lessin of the George Washington Medical Center (Fig. 42) and Dr D. F. Mahon of the City of Birmingham Public Health Department (Fig. 52). In addition Dr P. Fullerton and Professor G. W. Richter were both kind enough to allow us to use the originals of photographs which had already been published (Figs 43, 45 and 46). Miss B. M. Cornes prepared Fig. 4. To all these people we would like to extend our thanks.

Many of the other figures have been reproduced from published material and we are grateful to the original authors and the copyright holders for allowing us to use them. They include Academic Press Inc (Figs 31 and 32), the Air Pollution Control Association (Figs 12 and 14), the American Association for the Advancement of Science (Figs 5, 11, 46 and 47), the American Association of Pathologists and Bacteriologists (Fig. 45), the American Chemical Society (Figs 6, 7, 10 and 13), the American Medical Association (Fig. 15), the British Medical Association (Figs 20, 21, and 23–30), the Editor of the Lancet (Fig. 48), the Editor of the Journal of Neuropathology and Experimental Neurology (Figs 43 and 44), the Editorial Board of the Biochemical Journal (Fig. 19), the Elsevier Publishing Company (Fig. 9), Microfilms International Marketing Corporation (Figs 3, 8, 16 and 33–38) and the Wistar Press (Figs 17 and 18).

Contents

Introduction

THE CHANGING PATTERN OF LEAD POISONING

Few metals have a longer history of use by man than lead and there is none with a greater literature cataloguing its ill effects on those who come into contact with it. The number of deaths attributable to lead poisoning, however, has fallen during this century to a very low figure and accounts at most for no more than four or five cases annually. The notification of industrial cases to the Factory Inspectorate has shown a similar downward trend and there has been only one industrial fatality since 1950 (Figs 1 and 2, see p. 7).

This improvement in health standards has been accomplished at a time when the industrial use of lead has been on the increase. Far from becoming complacent about the situation a large body of opinion has expressed concern about the amount of lead being mobilized into the environment especially through the agency of leaded petrol. Lead poisoning is assuming what Hammond (1969) has called a new dimension and it is felt by some that the current levels of lead in the environment constitute a chronic threat to health, so that although the nature of the problem has changed its extent may be potentially greater than before.

DEFINITION OF TERMS

The terms lead absorption and lead poisoning are not used consistently everywhere, and it is convenient to define their use here. These definitions are elaborated from others given in an earlier publication (Waldron, 1971).

Lead Absorption

Lead absorption is the process whereby an individual takes up lead from the environment by whatever means, and at whatever stage he is in his development.

Lead Poisoning

Lead poisoning may be metabolic or clinical. Metabolic poisoning may be said to be present when it is possible to detect alterations in metabolism which are the result of lead absorption. Clinical lead poisoning is diagnosed when the absorbed lead produces signs or symptoms which are evident to the patient or his doctor. Metabolic poisoning may exist without clinical poisoning but not the converse.

Sub-clinical Poisoning

Recently the concept of sub-clinical lead poisoning has been elaborated and this may be defined as the production of morbidity or mortality without the appearance of the classical signs or symptoms of clinical lead poisoning.

Other Terms

Plumbism, saturnism and lead intoxication are all terms which are used as synonyms for clinical lead poisoning.

1 Lead in the Environment

I. THE NATURAL LEVELS OF LEAD IN THE ENVIRONMENT

The presence of lead in the earth's crust results in the natural mobilization of the metal into the environment. The average lead content of the earth's crust is 16 ppm (de Treville, 1964), acid rocks containing more than basic rocks in the ratio of 20:8. The average lead content of soil is also 16 ppm (Stubbs, 1972). As a consequence of its presence in soil and water, lead enters the food chain and becomes incorporated into plant and animal tissue. An assessment of the degree of natural contamination of the environment has been made by Patterson (1965),[1] according to whom there are six significant sources of natural lead in the atmosphere. These are, in order of decreasing importance:

silicate dusts from natural soils
volcanic halogen aerosols
volcanic silicate smokes
forest fire smokes
aerosolic sea salts
meteoric smoke.

The estimated contribution of each of these to the natural atmospheric lead content is shown in Table 1 and the total is in the range 0·0005–0·0006 $\mu g/m^3$. Some of the atmospheric lead ultimately finds its way into the sea and the estimate for the natural lead concentration in fresh surface waters is approximately 0·0005 ppm.

---

[1] Patterson uses the term "natural" to refer to the lead levels in plant or animal tissue and in the environment, which are equivalent to those which prevail solely as the result of natural mobilization. He uses the term "contaminated" when referring to lead levels which have been elevated above natural levels by man-made mobilization. To designate blood lead levels which are above the (estimated) natural range but are not associated with frank illness, he uses the term "typical". This nomenclature is followed throughout this book.

Table 1

Estimated atmospheric lead concentrations from natural sources

Source	Concentration $\mu gPb/m^3$
Silicate dust	5×10^{-4}
Volcanic halogen aerosols	3×10^{-5}
Volcanic silicate smoke	6×10^{-6}
Forest fire smoke	6×10^{-6}
Aerosolic sea salts	1×10^{-6}
Meteorites and meteoric smoke	2×10^{-9}

From Patterson (1965)

Extending his argument still further, Patterson has calculated the natural daily intake of lead, both from the diet, through food and drinking water, and from the atmosphere and has also given figures for the expected concentration in organic materials. His estimate of the natural body burden is 2 mg Pb/70 kg body weight and of natural blood concentration, 0·0025 ppm (Table 2).

Table 2

Natural lead concentration in organic materials and natural lead intake

Lead content of whole plants	0·4 ppm
Lead content of whole animals	0·03 ppm
Lead content in human food	0·01 ppm
Ingestion from food	20 μg/day
Ingestion from water	0·5 μg/day
Ingestion from air	0·01 μg/day
Total body burden/ 70 kg body weight	2·0 mgm
Blood lead concentration	0·0025 ppm

From Patterson (1965)

Patterson's figures are, of course, speculative but have received some confirmation from the analysis of deep ocean waters, which represent uncontaminated water, and from air samples taken from areas where contamination is minimal. The lead concentration in deep sea waters of the Atlantic, Mediterranean and Pacific oceans, is well below Patterson's estimate of natural levels (Tatsumoto and Patterson, 1963; Chow and Patterson, 1966) although surface waters contain significantly higher concentrations of lead (see Section III). Atmospheric lead concentrations from Greenland (0·005 $\mu g/m^3$) and Novya Zemlya (0·0002) are also consistent with Patterson's figures whilst the concentrations found on the White Mountain and Laguna Mountain in California at sites above the thermal inversion zone were found to have a mean value of 0·008 $\mu g/m^3$ (Murozumi *et al.*, 1969; Egorov *et al.*, 1970; Chow *et al.*, 1972).

II. MAN-MADE MOBILIZATION IN HISTORIC TIMES

Lead was one of the seven metals of antiquity and has accompanied the Euro-Asian and the American civilizations, in part at least, since their beginning. Lead does not occur in an elemental state but its sulphide ore, galena (PbS), is common and was probably first used in antiquity as an eye-paint and for making into ornaments (Aitcheson, 1960). The discovery of metallic lead may have resulted from the accidental dropping of galena onto the camp fire and this may have been the original smelting furnace (Gowland, 1912). Lead oxide is readily reducible at temperatures below 800°C which are easily achieved in a domestic fire burning either dry wood or charcoal. In the process, galena is reduced to its oxide which then reacts further with unchanged galena to give metallic lead.

$$2PbO + PbS = 3Pb + SO_2$$

The lead produced would melt in the fire and collect in the ashes.

There is both written and archeological evidence that lead was in widespread use throughout the ancient civilizations. In the tribute lists of the Pharoah Thutmosis III (*ca* 1500 B.C.) there is mention of captured lead and his armies are known to have brought it home from Mesopotamia. Lead was used for many purposes by the Egyptians, including the making of human and animal figures, amulets, sinkers for fishing nets, rings, dishes, trays and other ornaments. It was also used as a core for bronze statuettes and bronze weights were often filled with lead. Eye-paints were used extensively and frequently contained lead compounds as pigments (Partington, 1935). The tribute lists of the pharoahs show that the peoples of the eastern border of the Mediterranean used lead before the time of the exodus of the Hebrews from Egypt. It is mentioned in the Old Testament and the process of cupellation by which silver was won from argentiferous galena is alluded to in the book of Jeremiah.

In the Mediterranean cultures, lead was frequently used in building work. In stone buildings molten lead was poured into the joints between the ashlars. Alternatively, the stones might be cramped with iron bars which were inserted into holes and held in place with lead. In the Mausoleum of Halikamossos the stone which closed the tomb chamber was fastened with a bronze pin. The pin and the ingle on the door frame were held in the stone with lead. Bands of lead were used where today iron wire would be utilized and in some instances, ceramic wine casks were hooped with lead instead of iron. The metal was also used in fishing and shipbuilding, as sinkers for nets, in anchor construction, as plummets for measuring depths of water beneath the keel, and in sheet form to protect the bottom of ships against worms. It also had a use in warfare as sling shot and often soldiers in beseiged garrisons tried to overthrow the battering rams of their aggressors with lead weights. Wrestlers in the arena fastened pieces of lead onto the leather thongs wound around their hands and arms to make their blows more punishing. The softness of the metal made it suitable for writing, both as a pencil and as a slate in which letters could be easily scratched. Many such slates have come down from antiquity. In many cases they are "curse slates" smuggled into the coffin or the grave of an enemy in order to produce a visitation of demons and evil spirits upon the dead. Lead also served as a material from which to fashion tickets, visiting cards, trade marks and coins.

In the ancient civilizations of India, lead was used for making amulets and weights for looms, and there is evidence for its use in China—where it was used as a stimulant in the court of the Emperors—and in pre-Columbian Mexico where a lead amulet dating from that period has been discovered.

The importance of lead in pre-Roman times, however, was in its association with silver. In the early centuries of the third millenium, tribes living on the Black Sea coast near to Pontus in Asia Minor discovered the important process of cupellation. This involved oxidizing the silver-bearing ore to litharge (PbO) which was absorbed onto a bulk material such as bone-ash, leaving behind the unaltered noble metal. So important was the recovery of silver from lead-ore that lead mines were often called silver mines. The amount of silver in galena varied considerably. In British galena the amount was not great, but some of the mines of Asia Minor produced lead ore yielding about 600 oz silver/ton (Tylecote, 1964) whilst the infamous Laurion mine on which the wealth of Athens was founded, yielded about 130 oz/ton (Aitcheson, 1960).

With the development of the Roman Empire, lead emerged from the background and assumed a dominant role in its technology (Boulakia, 1972). The Romans took lead from several countries of the Empire, Gaul, Britain and Germany, but chiefly from Spain, which had earlier supplied lead to Carthage. One of their shelf furnaces used for smelting lead has been found at Ailes-sur-Tech on the eastern border of the Pyrenees. It was completely underground and measured 3·2 × 2·5 metres. The walls were made of a fireproof mixture and the furnace was charged with alternate layers of lead ore and wood. The melted lead was carried away from the furnace via a channel in the ground.

The Romans' lead technology was impressive, and by far the largest part of their lead consumption went to make their extensive aquaducts and water mains. The aquaducts were lined with lead to caulk them and one such lining has been preserved on the Pont du Gard in the Rhône valley. There is scarcely any locality which was not equipped with leaden pipes, although earthenware water pipes were also widely used. The lead piping was produced by bending three-metre lengths of sheet lead around a core and soldering the seam. Piping was produced in seventeen standard sizes varying in diameter from 2·2 to 22·8 cm. Water supply charges were calculated on the diameter of the pipes supplying the household but the resourceful Romans found a way to cheat the magistrate by fixing a discharge mouth to the outlet which was of a different diameter from the supply pipe. The lengths of piping were joined together by fitting an end into a socket joint of the preceding pipe and fastening it with putty.

The large water reservoirs of the public supply systems were lead-lined and this practice was followed by the Greeks although they did not make use of leaden water pipes. They did, however, collect rain water from lead-lined rooves and often stored olive oil in lead-lined vessels.

Lead was also used extensively in cooking (Hofmann, 1885). The bronze pots of the Greeks and Romans gave a bitter taste to food cooked in them but it was found that a lead lining prevented this spoilation and also sweetened the food. Wine and sapa, which was used extensively as a sweetener, were prepared in lead-lined pots specifically because of this sweetening quality. These practices lead to considerable contamination of food and drink (Hofmann, 1883), and Gilfillan (1965) has advanced a theory that the Fall of the Roman Empire was largely due to endemic lead poisoning.

During the first two centuries of the present era it has been estimated that the consumption of lead reached a maximum of 4 kg/capita/year, a figure approaching the rate of consumption in the present-day United States of America which stands at about 6 kg/capita/year (Patterson, 1965).

Following the Fall of Rome in the fourth century, the use of lead declined and remained at a low level for about six hundred years. After the ninth century, however, lead ores began to be mined in eastern Germany. The practice of adulterating wine with lead and its salts became widespread, and was banned by an Imperial Law in 1498. The practice continued in spite of this edict and endemics of lead colic were by no means infrequent. In his classic tract on the Devonshire Colic, Sir George Baker (1767) traced the illness to cider contaminated with lead and he also gave a vivid account of the earlier continental endemics (Baker, 1768). Lead colic was common in colonial America (McCord, 1953), mainly due to the distillation of rum in leaden worms, and to the use of pewter and glazed earthenware with a high lead content.

III. PRESENT-DAY ENVIRONMENTAL LEVELS

The uses to which lead is now put are many and various (Ziegfield, 1964; Patterson, 1965; Stubbs, 1972). Table 3 compares the American and

Table 3

Principle uses of lead in 1970

	United States of America[a]		Great Britain[b]	
	tonnes	%	tonnes	%
Cables	50 772	3·7	60 000	17·2
Batteries	283 451	20·8	49 000	14·0
Sheet and Pipe	38 939	2·9	53 000	15·2
Foil	5 521	0·4	400	0·1
Collapsible tubes	10 913	0·8	2 000	0·6
Solder	69 707	5·1	14 000	4·0
Other metallic uses	213 384	15·7	50 000	14·0
Battery oxides	310 002	22·8	46 000	13·2
Lead alkyls	278 505	20·5	40 000	11·5
White lead	5 936	0·4	3 000	0·9
Other oxides and compounds	93 423	6·9	32 000	9·2
TOTAL	1 360 552	100·0	349 000	100·0

[a] Minerals Year Book (1970)
[b] Stubbs (1972)

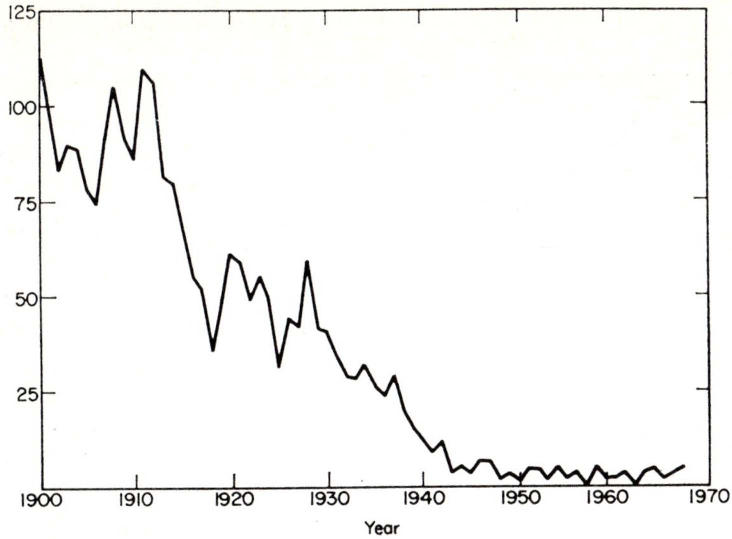

FIG. 1. Annual number of deaths from lead poisoning 1900–1966. Note that after 1966 the disease is no longer classified separately as a cause of death.

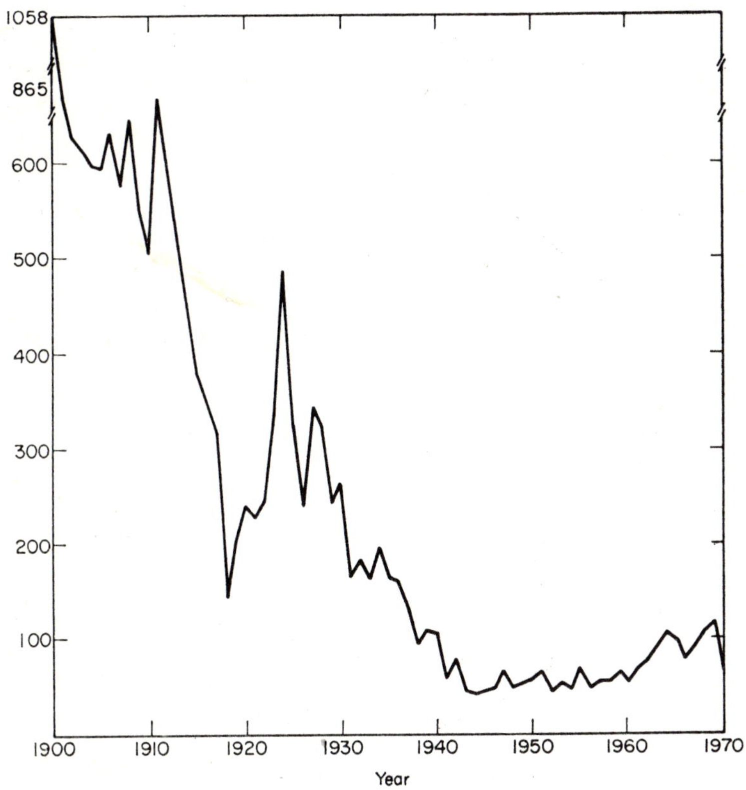

FIG. 2. Annual notifications of industrial lead poisoning to the Factory Inspectorate 1900–1970.

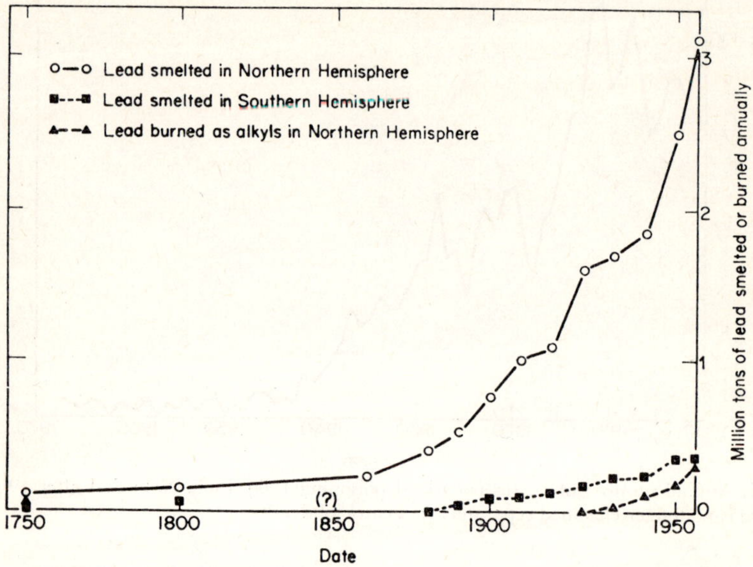

FIG. 3. World lead smelter and lead alkyl production since 1750. Note the difference in the consumption in the two hemispheres. Reproduced with permission from Murozumi *et al.* (1969).

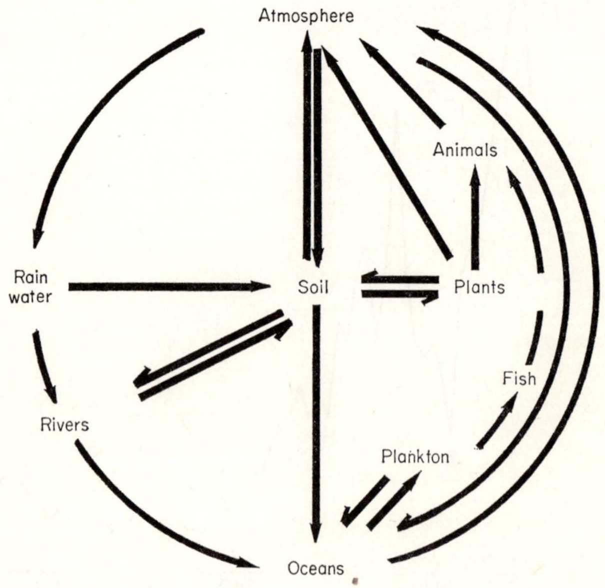

FIG. 4. The circulation of lead in the environment.

British usage in 1970. In America most lead is used to make batteries, battery oxides and lead alkyls. In Great Britain these do not have prime importance, but whereas metallic uses, with the exception of battery making, are now decreasing, the manufacture of lead alkyls has increased, from 27,000 tonnes in 1960 and 37,000 in 1965 to 40,000 in 1970. The manufacture of battery oxide is increasing at the same rate as battery production and all three rises reflect an increase in motor-car production.

The use of lead has increased considerably during this century and is continuing to do so (Fig. 3), and it is important to assess the effect which this increased mobilization of lead is having on environmental lead levels.

The circulation of lead in the ecosphere is shown diagramatically in Fig. 4.

A. Atmospheric Lead Concentrations

In the last few years considerable data have been produced, some of which are shown in Table 4. The data show that the level of lead in urban areas exceeds that in rural areas and values are greater during the day than at night (Jost *et al.*, 1972). There is also a very considerable seasonal variation (Chow and Earl, 1970; Bowman *et al.*, 1972, Lawther *et al.*, 1972). Ventilation in cities is determined by the formation of horizontal air currents beneath inversion layer ceilings. These ceilings are higher in summer than in winter, which means that the city air chamber is less in winter than summer and hence the atmospheric lead concentration is raised (Fig. 5; Patterson, 1971). When atmospheric concentrations are expressed as an average throughout the year, these are found to be relatively constant (Bowman *et al.*, 1972). See Table 5.

Within cities, the atmospheric lead concentration is also a function of traffic density. With increasing traffic flow the ambient lead levels rise (Table 6). The increase in lead concentrations is not constant, but is inversely proportional to the distance from the roadway along which the traffic passes (Fig. 6). The particle size of the lead aerosol decreases with increasing distances from the roadway (Fig. 7) indicating a settling-out of the large particles close to the road (Daines *et al.*, 1970).

The size of the population of a city also determines to some extent the level of lead found in the air (Table 7). This may relate to the number of cars and to the pollution from factories and domestic coal-burning fires. Meteorological conditions are obviously important in determining the levels of lead found at a single sampling point, and this is shown in

Table 4

Atmospheric lead concentration in different sites

Location	Area sampled	Lead conc. μg/m³	Authors
N. Central Pacific Ocean		0·0010	Chow *et al.* (1969)
S. Indian Ocean		0·0010	Egorov *et al.* (1970)
Oahu		0·0017	Jernigan *et al.* (1971)
Nova Zemlya		0·002	Egorov *et al.* (1970)
N. Indian Ocean		0·004	Egorov *et al.* (1970)
Greenland		0·005	Murozumi *et al.* (1969)
California	White and Laguna Mts	0·008	Chow *et al.* (1972)
St Moritz		0·02–0·1	Jost *et al.* (1972)
Taunus Observatory		0·06–0·6	Jost *et al.* (1972)
Warsaw		0·09	Jaworoswki (1963)
Cambridge, Mass.		0·1–2·2	Liniger *et al.* (1966)
California	Remote mountains	0·12	Calif. Public Health Dept. (1967)
Alaska University		0·19	Winchester *et al.* (1967)
Edinburgh		0·19	Ireland (1972)
Bristol		0·22	Ireland (1972)
Tula	After ban on leaded petrol	0·24	Dubrovskaya (1960)
Glasgow		0·25	Ireland (1972)
Leeds		0·39	Ireland (1972)
Cardiff		0·40	Ireland (1972)
Berlin	Quiet streets	0·4–0·5	Lahmann and Möller (1967)
Hamburg		0·4–7·5	Szadkowski and Lehnert (1972)
Wolverhampton		0·51	Ireland (1972)
Sheffield		0·52	Ireland (1972)
Liege	Urban zone	0·6–0·9	Rondia and de Graeve (1972)
Middlesborough		0·66	Ireland (1972)
Manchester		0·71	Ireland (1972)
Tipton		0·71	Ireland (1972)
West Bromwich		0·71	Ireland (1972)
Stoke-on-Trent		0·89	Ireland (1972)
Otaru City		0·95–3·00	Endo *et al.* (1968)
Cincinnatti		1·4	United States Public Health Service (1965)

Table 4 (*contd.*)

Location	Area sampled	Lead conc. μg/m³	Authors
Tula	Before ban on leaded petrol	1·4	Dubrovskaya (1960)
Zurich	Near traffic	1·4	Eidg. Gesundheits Amt. (1961)
Liege	Industrial zone	1·4–2·4	Rondia and De Graeve (1972)
Philadelphia		1·6	United States Public Health Service (1965)
Hamburg	Quiet street	2·0	Hettche (1964)
Dushanbe	Arterial road	2·0	Berdyev *et al.* (1967)
Niigata City	City crossroads	2·02–3·81	Kifune *et al.* (1970)
London	St Bart's Med. College	2·1–2·8	Lawther *et al.* (1972)
Milan		2·4–7·4	Giubileo (1967)
Vienna	Winter	2·6	Hartl and Resch (1972)
Vienna	Summer	2·9	Hartl and Resch (1972)
German cities: Mullheim, Düsseldorf, Neuss, Wuppertal, Duisberg	Quarter mile from traffic	3·2	Heller and Kettner (1968)
London	Fleet Street	3·2	Waller *et al.* (1965)
Paris		3·25–9·8	Truffert *et al.* (1966)
Warwick	Busy street	3·5	Bullock and Lewis (1968)
Berlin	Busy street	3·8	Lahmann and Möller (1967)
Chelyabinsk		3·86	Dubrovskaya (1960)
New York	2–75 m from traffic	4·1	Colucci *et al.* (1969)
Los Angeles	Central city	4·3–6·6	Colucci *et al.* (1969)
Paris	Central streets	4·8	Lebbe (1965)
Detroit	5–150 m from traffic	4·8	Colucci *et al.* (1969)
Fairbanks		6·0	Winchester *et al.* (1967)
Genoa		7·36–14·2	Petrilli *et al.* (1966)
Los Angeles	4–20 m from traffic	7·6	Colucci *et al.* (1969)

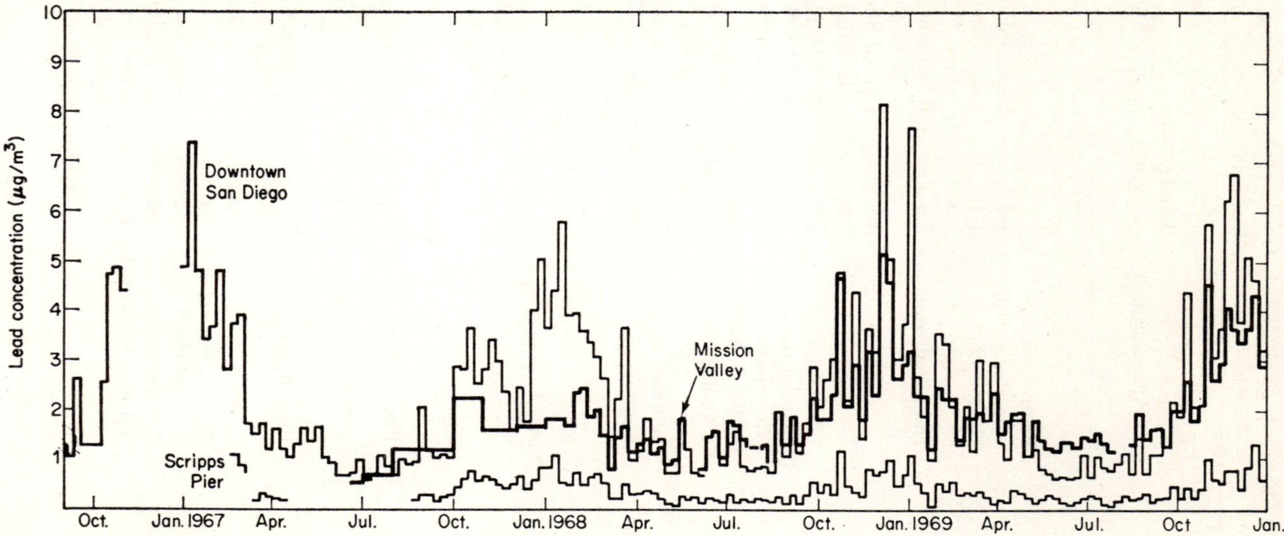

FIG. 5. Concentration of lead in the air near San Diego, California, showing seasonal variation. Reproduced with permission from Chow and Earl (1970).

Table 5

Daily average of atmospheric lead concentration in Berkeley, California

Year	Mean concentration $\mu gPb/m^3$
1963	2·8
1964	2·8
1965	3·0
1966	3·0
1967	3·1
1968	3·2
1969	3·0
1970	2·9

From Bowman *et al.* (1972)

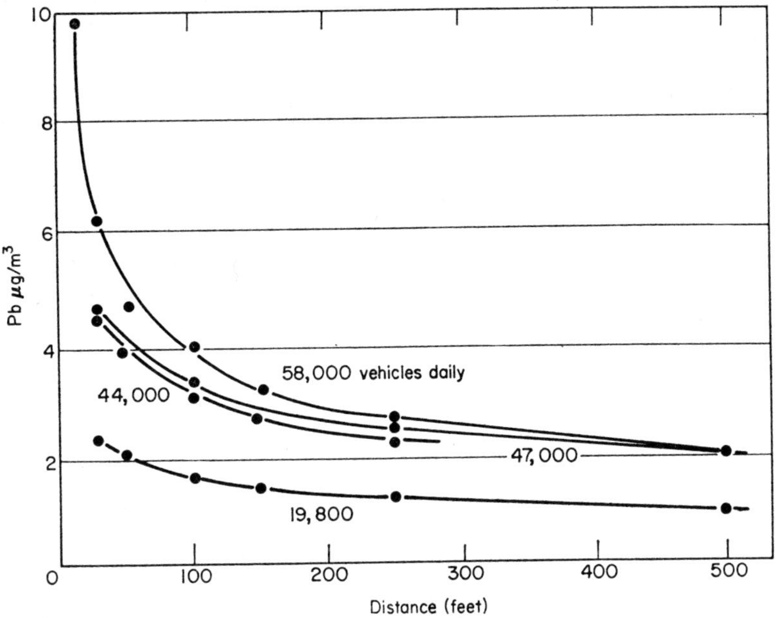

Fig. 6. Atmospheric lead concentrations as a function of traffic density and distance from the highway. Reproduced with permission from Daines *et al.* (1970).

Table 6

Variation of mean atmospheric lead concentration with increasing traffic density

Traffic volume cars/hour	Mean concentration $\mu gPb/m^3$
500	4·6
820	4·8
2150	7·6

From Public Health Service Publication 999-Ap-12 (1965)

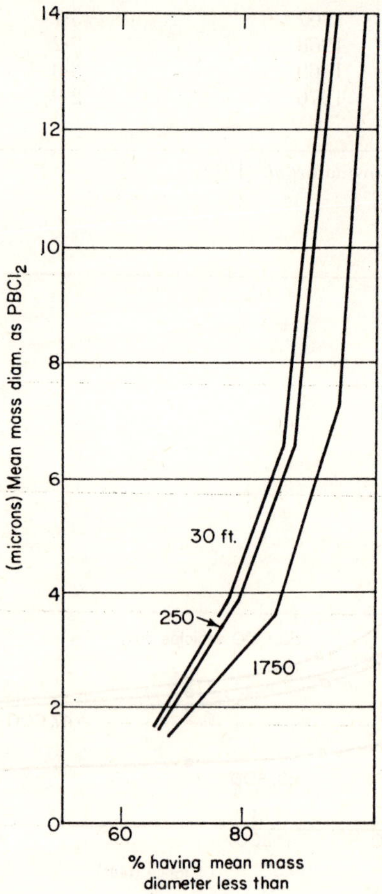

FIG. 7. Relationship of particle size of airborne lead to distance from the highway. Reproduced with permission from Daines *et al.* (1970).

Table 7

Variation of mean atmospheric lead concentration with increasing population

City population million	Mean concentration μgPb/m^3
<0·5	0·65
0·5–2·0	1·00
2·0	3·20

From Stanford Research Institute (1956)

Table 8. When a site is close to a highway, changes in wind direction can affect dramatically the concentration of lead found at the site (Table 9). Blemel (1967) has developed an equation for predicting levels of atmospheric lead concentration emanating from car exhausts which utilizes traffic patterns, wind direction and an inverse logarithmic function of wind speeds for its parameters. Finally, it has been found that lead concentrations vary according to the vertical height above street level (Table 10).

Table 8

The effect of meteorological condition on atmospheric lead concentrations

Sample	Meteorological conditions	Mean concentration μg/m^3
1	Weak westerly winds,	2·04
2	strong temperature	2·31
3	inversion, low visibility	3·32
4		3·70
5		3·30
6		0·68
7	Brisk easterly winds, no	1·33
8	clouds, good visibility	0·45
9		1·84
10		1·66
11		0·39

From Moyers *et al.* (1972)

Table 9

Relationship of wind direction to atmospheric lead concentrations at three distances from a highway supporting 47,000 cars daily

Wind direction	Mean concentration at feet from highway μg Pb/m^3		
	30	75	125
East to south	1·00	1·08	0·71
North to west	5·31	4·23	3·54

From Daines *et al.* (1970)

Table 10

Variation of atmospheric lead concentrations with increasing height of the sampling station above street level. The table also shows diurnal variation

Height	6 m	12 m	34 m	
Mean	3·2 ± 1·6	3·1 ± 1·7	2·0 ± 1·1	Day time
Concentration μgPb/m^3	2·4 ± 0·9	2·0 ± 1·1	1·3 ± 0·6	Night time

From Jost *et al.* (1972)

It is clear from these considerations that great care must be exercised when comparing data from different studies. The data do bear out the hypothesis, however, that atmospheric levels rise according to the proximity of the sample to cities. Patterson has over-simplified the situation by suggesting the following approximations for air lead concentrations ($\mu g/m^3$):

North polar region $< 0{\cdot}0005$
Central ocean regions 0·001
United States countryside 0·05
United States cities 2.

Nevertheless, there is sufficient evidence to show that the level of lead in the atmosphere is greatly in excess of Patterson's natural level or of the baseline level of 0·008 $\mu g/m^3$ recently suggested by Chow *et al.* (1972).

B. Hydrosphere

Lazrus and his colleagues (1970) suggest that the atmospheric lead aerosol remains in a soluble form as the halide or sulphate. The very insoluble lead dioxide is thought to react with atmospheric sulphur dioxide to produce the sulphate which is soluble at low atmospheric concentrations. Concentrations of lead halide, however, are likely to be very low since most of it changes into other lead species (Ter Haar and Bayard, 1971). (See Section V, p. 31.) A considerable fraction of the lead aerosol is washed out by rainfall at heights from one to ten kilometres (Hicks *et al.*, 1966) and the residence time of lead in the atmosphere is from two to thirty-three days (Lehmann and Sittkus, 1959; Burton and Stewart, 1960; Fry and Menon, 1962; Francis *et al.*, 1970). The relative effectiveness of washing out compared with dry sedimentation and impaction in removing lead from the atmosphere was studied by Atkins and Kruger (1968). Their experiments were conducted at Palo Alto, where the rainfall averages thirteen inches a year. They found the mean concentration of lead in rain collected near the freeway was 0·18 mg per litre whilst at the city outskirts it was 0·04 mg per litre. The authors considered that the higher concentration found near the freeway was due to the aggregation of the lead particles in the atmosphere. Their overall conclusion was that rainfall and dry sedimentation are the major factors for removing lead from the atmosphere, and that ten per cent or more of lead reaching the ground in areas removed from major roadways was carried by rain water.

High levels of lead in rain water collected near a busy main traffic artery in Cincinatti were reported by Ettinger (1966). Five of twelve samples showed lead in excess of 0·1 mg per litre and one sample had a value of 0·49 mg per litre. It was felt, however, that contamination with dust could not be ruled out. A significant correlation between the concentration of lead in rain water and the sale of gasoline in the area sampled was noted by Lazrus and his colleagues (1970). They sampled rain at 32 locations in the United States over a period of 4 months. The mean concentration was 0·034 mg Pb per litre and the rank correlation coefficient between the lead concentration and sale of petrol was 0·55 ($p < 0{\cdot}5$).

Meteorological conditions affect the concentration of lead found in rain water, however. Ter Haar *et al.* (1967) found that slow, even rainfall was more effective in removing lead from the atmosphere than brisk showers although rain collected in thunderstorms did sometimes contain a high concentration of lead (Table 11). They concluded that rain water contributed little to the total lead content of the soil and estimated that it amounted to only about 1 μg per cm per year.

The concentration of lead in snow shows similar variations to that in rain water as might be expected. Schroeder and Balassa (1961) determined lead in snow in different sites in Brattleboro Retreat. On an open

Table 11

Relation of lead content of rain water to type of rainfall

Location	Precipitation (type)	Pb, μg/litre
Western Michigan	R	27·5
	R	29·2
	S	6·2
	TS	6·5
Argonne	R	44·3
	S	4·0
	S	4·6
	S	6·3
	S	9·2
	S	10·6
	S	13·2
	TS	3·8
	TS	20·6
	TS	87·4

R = slow, even rain
S = showers (rapid)
TS = thunder storms
From Ter Haar *et al.* (1967)

lawn, 300 metres from a well-used road it was 0·00525 ppm, 3 metres from the street it was 0·012 ppm and on the street the concentration was 0·077 ppm in fresh and ploughed snow. Much higher levels than this were reported by Hamilton and Miller (1971) who found the concentration of lead in snow collected within 100 feet of streets and roads in Columbus, Ohio had a mean of 0·41 ppm and all but one of their twenty-seven samples exceeded the safe limit of 0·05 ppm set by the United States Public Health Service for lead concentration in drinking water.

Murozumi *et al.* (1969) have advanced evidence that the lead concentration in rainfall, and by inference in the atmosphere, has risen in recent times. They collected samples of snow and ice from locations in northern Greenland and the Antarctic. They found that the concentration of lead varied inversely with the geological age of the sample. The concentration in snow dating from 800 A.D. was less than 0·001 μg per kg rising to more than 0·2 μg per kg in recent snow. The concentration rose steeply after about 1750 (coinciding with the Industrial Revolution) and again after 1940 (coinciding with an increase in the use of lead alkyls in petrol) (Fig. 8).

The levels in Antarctic snows were less than those found in Greenland by a factor greater than ten. Before 1940 the concentration was below detection but has since risen to about 0·02 μg per kg. The differences found in the two hemispheres reflects the vastly greater use of lead in the northern as compared with the southern hemisphere.

Both the results and the conclusions of Murozumi and his colleagues were criticized by Mills (1971) who suggested that the increase in the snow lead after 1940 could be due to aircraft using Thule (150 miles distant from the sampling site) and Camp Century (50 miles distant).

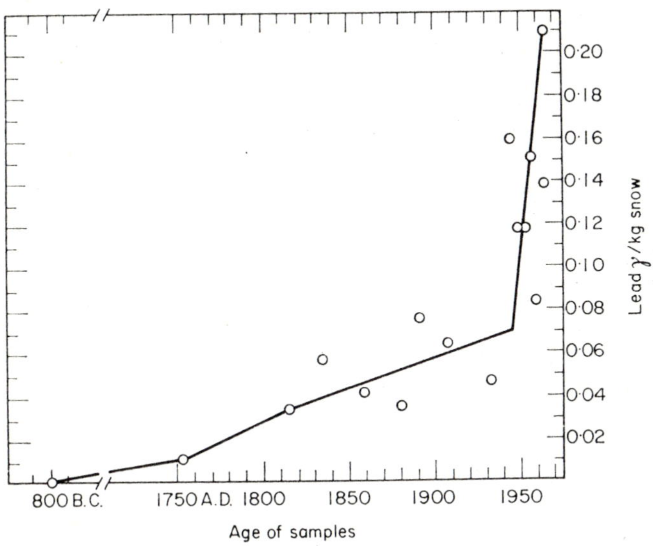

FIG. 8. Lead concentration profile in snow strata of northern Greenland. Reproduced with permission from Murozumi *et al.* (1969).

Bryce-Smith (1971b) has countered Mills's argument by stating that the greatest amounts of lead were found to be deposited in the snow in winter months when air traffic was lightest. Also, there was no gradient in lead concentration from the base to the collecting site, and in addition the collecting site was predominantly upwind from the base. Finally, Bryce-Smith noted that the major increase in the lead levels began about twenty years before the closer base was established. Jaworowski (1967) has found that lead concentrations in two Polish glaciers have increased by a factor of ten during the past century. The concentrations found in the latest ice-layers were so extremely high, however, (80–150 μg Pb per kg) that they may represent local, rather than general contamination.

Further proof of increasing atmospheric lead levels is to be gained from the analysis of sea water. Analysis of lead in oceanic sediments shows that about $1{\cdot}3 \times 10^{10}$ g of discharged lead entered the oceans per year, several million years ago, whilst measurement of lead in river water shows that some $2{\cdot}4 \times 10^{11}$ g of lead are currently entering the oceans (Patterson, 1971). Analysis of lead concentration profiles shows that young waters in the Pacific and Mediterranean Oceans contain an excess of lead compared with deep older layers (Tatsumoto and Patterson, 1963; Chow and Patterson, 1966). This pattern is not as striking in Atlantic waters (Fig. 9).

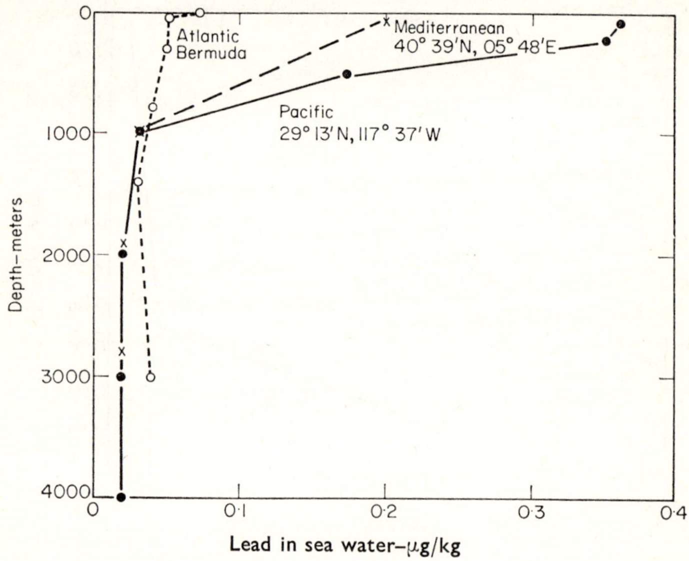

FIG. 9. Lead concentration profile in the oceans. Reproduced with permission from Chow and Patterson (1966).

C. Lead in Soil and Plants

The mean concentration of lead in the soil is of the order of 16 ppm, but varies considerably from one location to another (Table 12). High levels in the soil will be found in areas adjacent to lead smelters, in areas where lead arsenate has been used as a crop spray and in areas in close proximity to heavily used roads. In connection with the last point, the lead content of the soil is a function both of the closeness of the sample to the roadway and, for soils of similar composition, of the depth at which the sample is taken (Singer and Hanson, 1969; Motto *et al.*, 1970, Wiklander, 1970;

Table 12

The lead content of soil

Location	Lead content, ppm	Author
Russian soils	0·038–0·43	Sinyakova (1945) Vinogradov (1946, 1954)
India (Bengal and Calcutta)	0·04–0·06	Bagchi *et al.* (1940)
Mexico	0·07–8·0	Kehoe *et al.* (1933a)
Yucatan peninsula	0·08–25	Kehoe *et al.* (1933a)
Canadian soils	0·5–1,000	Warren and Delavault (1960)
East Africa	0·60	Chamberlain (1959)
Sarawac	1·20–30	Kehoe *et al.* (1933a)
Sarawac (river bed)	4·8	Kehoe *et al.* (1933a)
Podzol and forest soil	6–108	Wright *et al.* (1955)
New Jersey loam	13·9–95·7	Prince (1957)
Old residential soil	16·4–360	Cholak *et al.* (1961)
Near site of coal burning	17–3,000	Dunn and Bloxham (1932)
Soil near lead ore vein	20–10,000	Huff (1952)
French soil	207–261	Bertrand and Okada (1933)
Near site of coal burning	534–12,340	Manley (1937)
Near lead zinc smelter	778–40,175	Pakhotina (1958)

Kumashiro and Ogata, 1971) (Fig. 10). It has also been clearly shown that the contamination of vegetation growing along highways decreases the further they are from the road (Warren, 1959, 1961; Warren and Delavault, 1960; Cannon and Bowles, 1962; Kloke *et al.*, 1966; Rameau, 1968; Rühling and Tyler, 1968) (Fig. 11). This was confirmed by Motto *et al.* (1970) who studied the lead content of five crops grown in three fields at varying distances from highways. Those plants growing closest to the highways had the highest lead content. The distribution of lead in these plants was different from plants grown inside a greenhouse in leaded soils or sand. The crops in the fields contained most lead in the aerial parts whilst those grown in the leaded soils had most lead in the roots. These results indicated that plants may take up lead both by their leaves and roots but that relatively little translocation takes place within the plant, although Mitchell and Reith (1966) did observe translocation of lead from root to shoot in rye grass during the winter period.

These results are similar to those reported by Ter Haar (1970) who grew vegetables in greenhouses in filtered air and in unfiltered air with a lead content of 0·09 and 1·45 $\mu g/m^3$ respectively. He showed that in many instances the aerial parts of the plant growing in the unfiltered air had a higher lead content than those growing in filtered air indicating that some of the lead from the atmosphere was fixed by the shoots.

There is, in addition, botanical evidence that the concentration of atmospheric lead has risen over the last century. Rühling and Tyler measured the lead content in Swedish mosses and found an historical lead gradient. The concentration in mosses dating from 1860–1875 was about

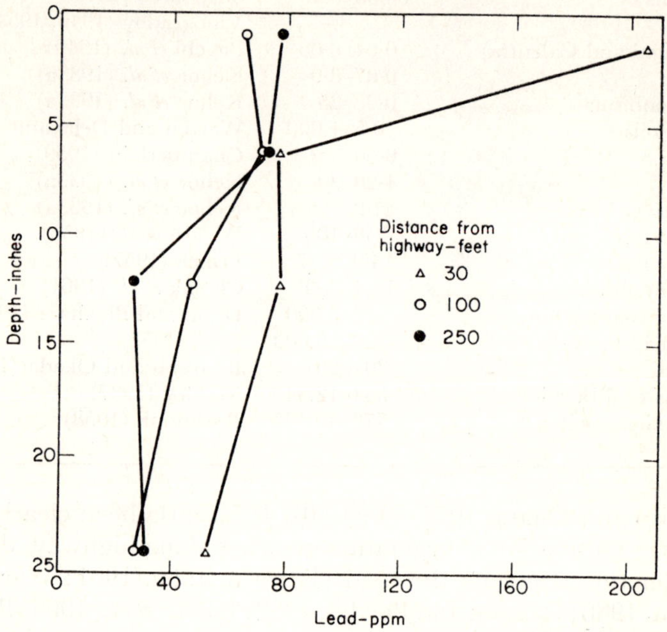

FIG. 10. Lead distribution with depth of soil. Reproduced with permission from Motto *et al.* (1970).

20 ppm and then more than doubled between 1875 and 1900. This value (40–50 ppm) remained constant until 1950 when there was an increase to present-day levels of 80–90 ppm (Rühling and Tyler, 1968). The first increase the authors related to increased industrialization with a concomitant rise in coal-burning, whilst the second rise correlated well with the rapid introduction of leaded petrol in Sweden. It has been found that the inner rings of trees contain less lead than the outer rings (Suchodoller, 1967; Ault *et al.*, 1970; Ter Haar, 1970) (Table 13).

From these data it appears that the trees have doubled their lead intake in the past thirty years. Ault *et al.* (1970) did not think this likely and suggested that it was more probable that lead was being translocated

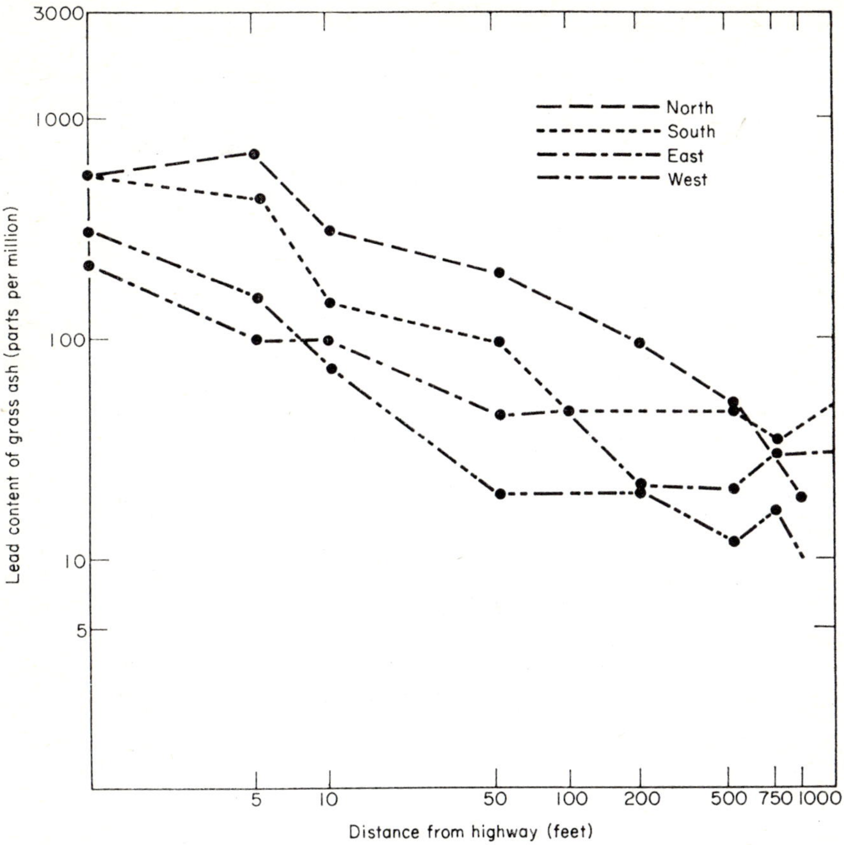

FIG. 11. Variation in lead content of grass alongside two major highways in the Denver, Colorado area. Reproduced with permission from Cannon and Bowles (1962).

from the xylem. Stewart (1966) has described a mechanism whereby toxic matter might be excreted from active cells and translocated along the radial ray cells of the woody part of the tree. Holtzman (1970), however, studied the distribution of ^{210}Pb in oak and hickory and found that the specific activity due to the isotope was constant in the outer rings but decayed towards the centre as predicted from the half-life of the isotope. The results were not as striking in the oaks as in the hickory but strongly suggested that there was no circulation of lead in hickory after twenty years and in oaks after five years. There is a curious anomaly in Ault *et al.*'s (1970) results in that the isotopic composition of lead in the wood is different from that found in the soil, bedrock, leaves and air. It is highly unlikely that the tree is "selecting" its lead source, and the most

Table 13

Variation of lead content with age of tree rings

	Concentration μgPb/gram	
Date	Red oak[a]	Elm[b]
1865–1870		0·16
1900–1910		0·12
1930–1937	0·16	
1940–1947		0·33
1950–1959		0·74
1951–1953	0·14	
1964–1966	0·34	

[a] From Ault *et al.* (1970)
[b] From Suchodoller (1967)

probable explanations are that either there was some error in the analysis or the sample was contaminated.

The effect of increased levels of lead in the atmosphere on the amount of lead taken in the diet is not altogether certain. A compilation of data is given in the Appendix and it will be seen that values do not appear to have risen during the past ten to forty years. Blokker (1972) concludes from his survey of the literature that the average intake of lead from food has not changed appreciably in the past three decades. It must be stressed, however, when comparing analytical results of thirty or forty years ago with those of the present, that the error in the methods used then was considerably greater than the more refined methods used nowadays and that older results are likely to be overestimates.

Lewis wrote in 1966 that the data obtained in his laboratory suggested that the level of lead in milk was higher than twenty to thirty years ago (0·04–0·05 mg per litre compared with 0·02–0·04 mg per litre). Rameau (1968) found that milk from cows eating roadside grass which had a lead content of 30–110 μg per g dry weight contained very little more lead than that from cows put into pasture far distant from roads. The concentrations found were 0·033 mg per litre against 0·026 mg per litre. Lanzola *et al.* (1972) found an increase in the lead content of milk produced in Pavia (Italy) during the last eight years.

In considering the pathways of lead from the air and soil to the gastro-intestinal tract of man via food, certain factors should be borne in mind.

Firstly, atmospheric lead will settle directly only on the aerial parts of plants and so is important only in relation to foods where the leaves and shoots are eaten. Secondly, as Jones and Clement (1972) have pointed out, there are a number of barriers which restrict the movement of lead. Thus, only a proportion of the total lead content of the soil is available for the plant, depending to some extent on the type of soil and the rooting habit. Soils with low organic content tend to promote uptake, whilst plants with shallow roots will have access to more lead than deep-rooted species. Of the lead which is absorbed by the plants, only a small proportion is transported to the shoots to become available to grazing animals, although atmospheric lead may settle onto the aerial parts, and of the lead taken in by grazing animals, a small fraction only is absorbed. Finally, of the lead which does pass into the body of the animals the great majority will be stored in the skeleton.

D. Street Dust

Analysis of the lead content of street dust was performed by Kaye and Reznikoff (1947) on dust collected in 1924 and 1934, that is before and after the introduction of leaded petrol. The number of samples analysed was small but the lead content of the dust was approximately fifty per cent greater in the later samples. Giubileo (1957) found the concentration of lead in the street dust of Milan was greatest in the city centre and decreased on peripheral streets, confirming the earlier work of Jecklin (1956) who found lead levels of dust in the centre of Basel up to forty times greater than in dust in a rural area. The values given by Giubileo were 1,360–2,360 ppm in central streets and 800 ppm in the others. Warren *et al.* (1971) found that the lead content of dust was a function of the volume of traffic as might be expected from a consideration of the relationship between lead-in-air concentrations and traffic. These high values have been confirmed. Högger (1971) for example, found a maximum of 2,040 ppm in Zurich whilst in Birmingham the highest value was $>$6,000 ppm (Stephens, 1972, personal communication). The proportion of lead in subfractions of different particle size of dust from the streets, increases with diminishing diameter (Rameau, 1972) and this may be significant in subsequent fractionation processes involving wind and rain.

House dust may contain high levels of lead, 20–30,700 ppm being found in a survey in Birmingham although there was considerable variation in samples taken within a short distance of each other (Stephens, 1972, personal communication).

IV. SOURCE OF LEAD IN THE ENVIRONMENT

Atmospheric lead may originate from a number of sources, including lead smelters, burning coal, refining lead scrap, the burning of materials containing lead, the recirculation by winds of lead in the soil and lead alkyls in petrol. The importance of each source has changed with time. During the early years of the Industrial Revolution lead smelters contributed considerable amounts of lead to the atmosphere due to the bad design of the furnaces and because smelting processes were inefficient. Although furnace design improved during the nineteenth century, it was not until the end of that century and the early part of the twentieth that the loss of fume from the smelters was reduced. Lead loss from the smelters has continued but has been further reduced so that it is now only about 0·06 per cent (compared with 0·5 per cent between 1880 and 1920 and an estimated two per cent from 1750–1880) (Murozumi *et al.*, 1969).

Present-day environmental lead contamination appears to come principally from leaded petrol (Table 14), although Jaworowski (1967) has suggested that the burning of coal contributes equally with lead alkyls in producing lead aerosol in the atmosphere. Murozumi *et al.* (1969), however, are of the opinion that coal burning has never been a significant contributor to atmospheric aerosol production even compared with the output from lead smelters in the 1930s, and they consider that Jaworowski arrived at his conclusion by overestimating the lead content of coal (17 ppm generally accepted) and the amount of coal converted to fine aerosol.

A technique for tracing the source of environmental lead is the determination of its isotopic ratio. Elemental lead is composed of four stable isotopes; ^{204}Pb, ^{206}Pb, ^{207}Pb, ^{208}Pb. ^{206}Pb, ^{207}Pb and ^{208}Pb are produced by the radioactive decay of ^{238}U, ^{235}U and ^{232}Th and have half-lives of 4·5, 0·7, 14×10^9 years respectively. ^{204}Pb has no radioactive progenitor. The isotopic ratio of lead ores from different sites has been studied in detail (Russell and Farquhar, 1960; Brown, 1962). Each ore has a unique isotopic composition which is a function of the geological age of the associated host rocks (Table 15). By studying the isotopic ratios of environmental lead it is possible to trace the ore from which it came. A comparison of the isotopic ratios of lead in coal, petrol, smelter ash and so on with that of atmospheric lead points to the contributing contaminator.

A number of studies of this kind have now been reported. Chow concludes from his work that atmospheric lead derives overwhelmingly from lead alkyls added to petrol (Chow and Johnston, 1965; Chow and Earl,

Table 14

Date	10^5 tons of lead smelted/year	Fraction converted to aerosols (%)	Tons of lead aerosols produced/year from smelters ($\times 10^3$)	10^5 tons of lead burned as alkyls/year	Fraction converted to aerosols (%)	Tons of lead aerosols produced/year from alkyls ($\times 10^3$)	Total tons of lead aerosols produced/year ($\times 10^3$)
1753	1	2	2	—	—	—	2
1815	2	2	4	—	—	—	4
1933	16	0·15	8	0·1	40	4	10
1966	31	0·06	2	3	40	100	100

From Murozumi *et al.* (1969)

Table 15

Isotopic composition of lead in major lead ores

	District	Host rock age	Pb^{206}/Pb^{204}	Pb^{206}/Pb^{207}	Pb^{206}/Pb^{208}
Australia	Broken Hill	Pre-Cambrian	16·07	1·037	0·4465
	Mt Isa	Pre-Cambrian	16·10	1·037	0·4464
Canada	NWT (Pine Point)	Ordovician	18·47	1·166	0·4792
	B.C. (Bluebell)	Cambrian	17·60	1·127	0·4738
	(North Star)	Pre-Cambrian	16·70	1·060	0·4535
	(Sullivan)	Pre-Cambrian	16·66	1·069	0·4578
	N.B. (Brunswick $\neq$ 12)	Ordovician	18·39	1·160	0·4770
	Newfoundland (Buchans)	Ordovician	18·18	1·150	0·4770
Mexico	Taxco	Tertiary	18·84	1·191	0·4836
	Durango	Tertiary	18·82	1·193	0·4836
Peru	Cerro de Pasco	Miocene	18·86	1·200	0·4816
	Casapalca	Miocene	18·89	1·204	0·4824
	San Cristobal	Miocene	18·87	1·201	0·4824
Yugoslavia	Trepca	Tertiary	18·83	1·195	0·4796
United States of America					
Missouri	Mississippi Valley	Pennsylvanian	21·78	1·385	0·5342
Idaho	Bunker Hill	Pre-Cambrian	16·45	1·052	0·4525
	Sunshine	Pre-Cambrian	16·55	1·062	0·4497
Utah	Tintic	Tertiary	18·50	1·179	0·4744
Colorado	San Miguel	Tertiary	19·88	1·233	0·4979

From Chow (1971)

1970; Chow, 1971) (Fig. 12), an opinion endorsed by the National Academy of Science of America (1971) who stated that 98% of the air-borne lead traceable to specific sources comes from the combustion of leaded petrol. Ault *et al.* (1970) and Rabinowitz and Wetherill (1972) have shown that the lead in the air, soil and vegetation near freeways is isotopically similar to lead in petrol but at points distant from the free-ways, lead from other sources (coal and smelters) was identifiable (Fig. 13). Smelter emission might be detectable in vegetation up to twenty miles from its source.

Although lead aerosol is ubiquitous, the personal environment of any particular individual may include more important sources of lead, including leaded paints, leaded glaze on pottery and food and drink

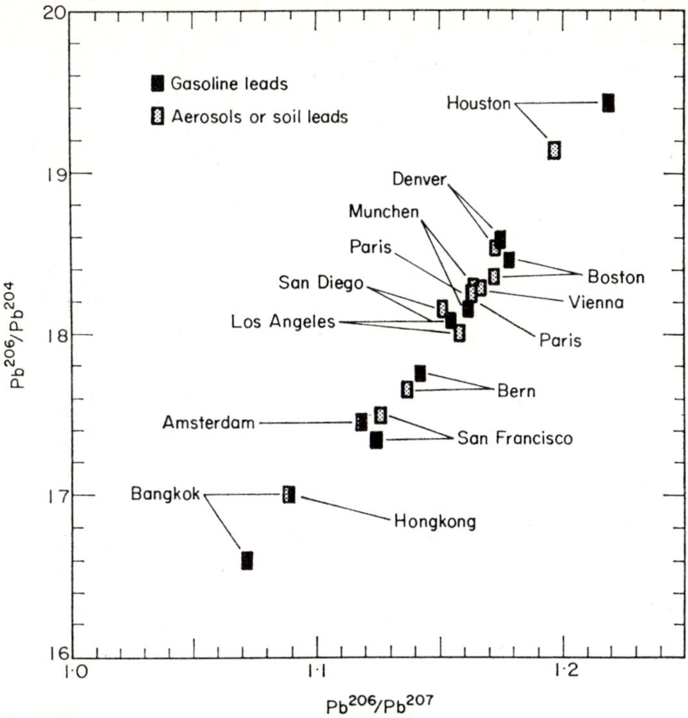

FIG. 12. Isotopic correlation between lead alkyl antiknock additives and pollutant leads. The dimension of the rectangle indicates measurement error. Reproduced with permission from Chow (1971).

contaminated in excess of the general levels, and cases of poisoning have been attributed to them all.

V. LEAD IN PETROL AND ITS EMISSION

Tetraethyl lead (TEL) was introduced as an anti-knock in petrol in February 1923 in Dayton, Ohio. It was distributed widely throughout the United States until May 1925 when it was withdrawn in most areas pending an investigation by the United States Public Health Service. Following the establishment of more stringent safety precautions in its manufacture and handling sales were continued in the summer of 1926 (Kehoe *et al.*, 1934). It was introduced into Great Britain during the 1930s but TEL was not manufactured there until 1940 (Cassells and Dodds, 1946). After 1960 tetramethyl lead (TML) became commercially

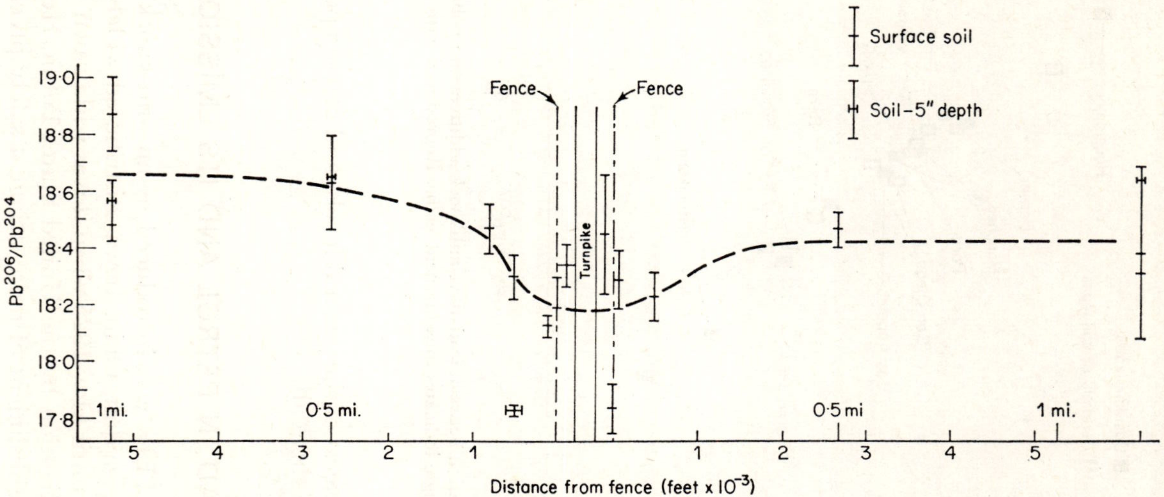

FIG. 13. Variations in lead isotopes in topsoil from a traverse across the New Jersey Turnpike. Mean ratio for lead from petrol = 18·3 ± 0·3; Mean ratio for lead from coal = 18·8 ± 0·2; Reproduced with permission from Ault *et al.* (1970).

available as an anti-knock agent. Compositions in current use as anti-knock agents contain lead-tetraethyl, -triethylmethyl, -diethyldimethyl, -ethyltrimethyl and -tetramethyl in proportions designed to give maximum overall efficiency.

The quantity of lead in petrol averages a little over two g/gallon (0·54 g/litre) in the United States of America (United States Public Health Service Publication, 1965) and in the United Kingdom the average is 0·46 g/litre, with higher grades containing more than lower grades (Institute of Petroleum Atmospheric Committee, 1971). In addition to lead alkyls, commercial anti-knock fluids contain 1,2-dihaloethanes as scavengers to reduce the accumulation of the decomposition products of the lead alkyls in certain critical areas of the combustion chamber. The most commonly used are ethylene dibromide and dichloride. During combustion the lead alkyls decompose and the resultant lead oxides react with the halogen scavengers to produce lead halides. The inorganic forms of lead produced and exhausted are PbCl.Br; α,β $NH_4Cl.2PbCl.Br$; $2NH_4Cl.PbCl.Br$; and minor amounts of $PbSO_4$; $PbO.PbCl.Br.H_2O$. If phosphorus additives are present in the petrol up to one-fifth of the lead in the exhaust gases may be present as $3Pb_3(PO_4)_2.PbCl.Br$ (United States Public Health Services Publication, 1965).

The lead halide compounds formed during combustion are very unstable. Within 18 hr 75 per cent of the bromide and 30–40 per cent of the chloride has been changed to lead carbonate, oxycarbonate and oxides. Studies of the composition of air taken near the roads shows a higher concentration of lead halides than air examined in a rural site distant from traffic confirming the breakdown of these compounds (Table 16). It has been suggested that the mechanism of breakdown of the lead halides in exhaust gas is photolytic (Pierrard, 1969); but since they also decompose when directly collected into light-proof bags, this seems most unlikely (Ter Haar and Bayard, 1971).

A variable amount of lead alkyl is emitted from the engine. Brief (1962) found that the ratio of organic to inorganic lead compounds in the exhaust gas was 0·1–0·53/0·33–3·1 mg per m^3 but Snyder (1967) found that organic lead accounted for only two to three per cent of the total. The quantity of organic lead emitted depends on the working temperature and running load of the car (Laveskog, 1971).

On occasions the carburettor temperature may be high enough to evaporate its contents, releasing lead alkyls into the atmosphere (Gartenmann, 1971). Most of the lead alkyls which escape, however, come from the crank-case (Laveskog, 1971).

Contributions to the total lead alkyl content in the atmosphere are made when car petrol tanks are filled when the vapour in the tank is

Table 16

Percentage of lead species in exhaust gas as a function of distance from traffic

Location	Lead compound											
	$PbCl_2$	$PbBr_2$	PbBrCl	Pb(OH)Cl	Pb(OH)Br	$(PbO)_2PbCl_2$	$(PbO)_2PbBr_2$	$(PbO)_2PbBrCl$	PbO_x	$(PbO)_2PbCO_2$	$PbCO_3$	Others
Near road	11·2	4·0	4·4	4·0	2·0	2·8	0·7	2·0	12·0	37·9	15·6	3·4
400 yd from road	10·5	0·7	0·6	8·8	1·1	5·6	0·3	0·6	25·0	21·3	14·6	10·9
Rural site	5·4	0·1	1·6	4·0	—	1·5	—	1·0	20·5	27·5	30·2	8·2

From Ter Haar and Bayard (1971)

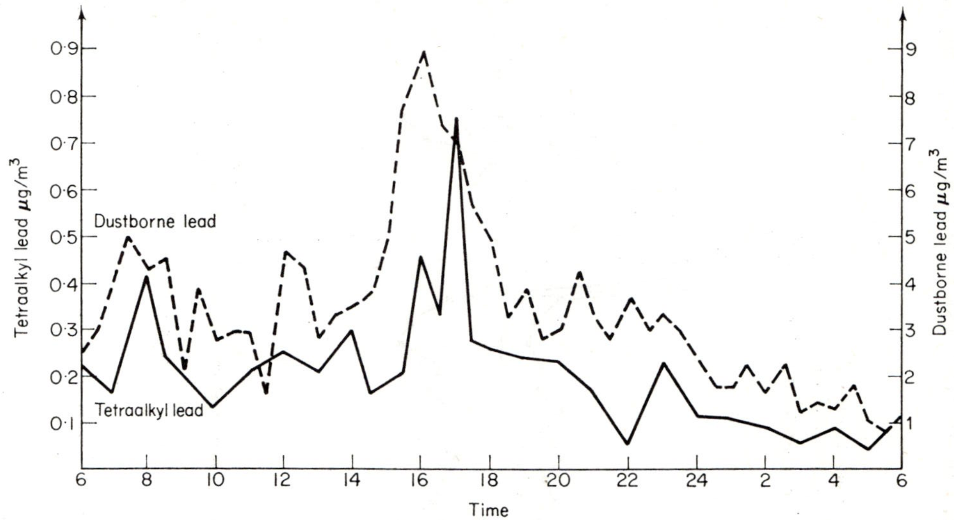

FIG. 14. Diurnal variation of tetra-alkyl lead and dust-borne lead in a major street in Stockholm. Reproduced with permission from Laveskog (1971).

displaced by petrol and high lead alkyl concentrations may be found in service stations (Zuliani *et al.*, 1966). The diurnal variation in atmospheric lead alkyl concentration closely parallels that of dustborne lead (Fig. 14) (Laveskog, 1971).

Of the lead which is put into the car in petrol, a quarter or more is retained as deposits on the exhaust system or in the lubricating oil and

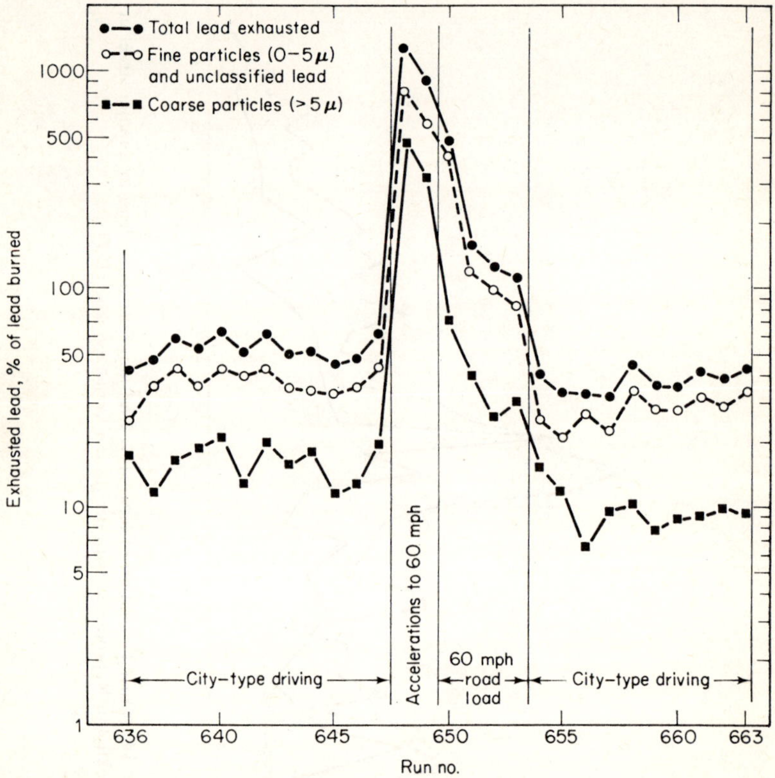

FIG. 15. Effects of different driving conditions on amount of lead emitted. Reproduced with permission from Hirschler and Gilbert (1964).

oil filters (Hirschler and Gilbert, 1964). Ter Haar *et al.* (1972) found that from 7–30 per cent of the lead consumed is exhausted and that 18 per cent of the lead burned is emitted as particles less than 5 μ mean maximal diameter (mmd). Mueller *et al.* (1963), however, found that only 10–20 per cent of burned lead was emitted in their experiments. The percentage of lead which is discharged is dependent upon the conditions under which the car is driven. Operations at high speeds with full-throttle acceleration discharge more lead than normal city driving at moderate speeds. Cold-cycle operation produces two to eight times more particulate matter in the exhaust system than hot-cycle operation (Ter Haar *et al.*, 1972). During any type of operation the exhaust system accumulates lead which may then flake off and be discharged into the atmosphere.

The particle size of the lead emitted covers a wide range. It has been estimated that more than half the lead exhausted in city driving is less than 8 μ, 40 per cent is less than 2 μ and 4–12 per cent is less than 1 μ. High speed driving increases the proportion of particles of large diameter emitted (Fig. 15) (Hirschler *et al.*, 1957; Mueller *et al.*, 1963; Hirschler and Gilbert, 1964).

VI. THE SIZE OF AIRBORNE PARTICLES

The mass median diameter of atmospheric lead particles has been determined by a number of workers and the results are shown in Table 17. It

Table 17

Particle size of airborne lead

Author	Mass median diameter, μ
Robinson and Ludwig (1964)	0·25
Lee *et al.* (1968)	0·18 (urban areas)
	0·48 (suburban areas)
Cholak *et al.* (1968)	0·30
Lundgren (1970)	0·20–0·90

may be seen that the mass median diameter is within the range at which considerable settling in the respiratory tract will occur. Recently direct electron microscope studies on airborne lead particles have shown that the larger particles are likely to be aggregates of smaller particles (Lawther *et al.*, 1972). This has been confirmed by Cerquiglini-Monteriolo and Funiciello (1972) who studied airborne particles having a diameter of 0·5 microns or more. Lead containing particles in this size range were found to be aggregates of lead and other material. The shape of these particles varies considerably, although about a half are spheroidal or ellipsoid.

VII. LEAD POISONING IN ANIMALS

Lead is the most common cause of accidental poisoning in domestic animals. The disease occurs most frequently in dogs and cattle and is related to their habit of chewing or licking objects indiscriminately. Dogs often develop plumbism as the result of chewing objects covered with lead-based paint or even eating metallic lead and the symptoms closely resemble those of distemper. Puppies are more commonly affected than older dogs because their eating habits are even less controlled (Zook *et al.*, 1969). Cattle have contracted lead poisoning from eating such diverse items as lead-based paint, used or discarded oil and oil filters, linoleum and storage batteries (Hammond *et al.*, 1956; Buck, 1970). Horses seldom develop lead poisoning from these sources but they seem more susceptible to the effects of chronic ingestion than cattle, with the result that they may develop symptoms of poisoning from grazing on lead-contaminated pastures whilst cattle grazing adjacent to them appear healthy (Larsen, 1969). Industrial fall-out, especially from lead smelters is a well-known source of contamination of grazing lands (Hammond and Aronsen, 1964; Kradel *et al.*, 1965; Ottoboni and Kahn, 1970) and in some regions the pollution has been so great that it is impossible to keep horses in the area (Gordon, 1968). Abortions have been reported in ewes grazing in areas around lead-mine and the lethal dose of lead is lower in pregnant than non-pregnant ewes (Allcroft and Blaxter, 1950).

Most of the lead is deposited directly onto the vegetation, not more than 15 μg/g of dry weight being translocated from the soil (Mueller and Stanley, 1970). Amounts greater than this can be considered as due to atmospheric fall-out. Contamination of the vegetation in the vicinity of smelters may be enormous—corn leaves growing 75 yards from a smelter were found to contain 3,200 μg/g (dry weight) (Hammond and Aronsen, 1964).

Vegetation growing alongside roadways has been found to be contaminated with lead from the settling-out of particles in the exhaust gases (Motto *et al.*, 1970) but the degree of contamination is apparently not sufficient to produce lead poisoning in grazing animals even for horses with their decreased tolerance (National Research Council, N.A.S., 1971).

Wild fowl are doubly unlucky, for not only may lead pellets kill them when fired by hunters, but the vast deposition of lead shot in their habitat (6,000 tons a year in the United States of America (Andrews and Longcore, 1969)) results in their ingestion of the pellets during their search for gravel. Lead poisoning in wildfowl is a serious problem (Andrews and

Longcore, 1969). Estimates of the number of birds which die from lead poisoning vary, but all are high (Munro and Solman, 1967; Bagley *et al.*, 1967; Richter and Schlatter, 1971) and in the United States of America it may be as many as one million per annum (Andrews and Longcore, 1969). The loss of birds is particularly serious because most die outside the hunting season and represent a loss of breeding stock.

The effects of lead on freshwater fish have been known since Carpenter's work on minnows (Carpenter, 1924, 1925 and 1926). Fish kept in cages in a river passing through an old lead mining area remained well until a period of heavy rain, after which they died. It was found that the concentration of lead in the river had increased from a value which was unrecordable to 0·3–0·4 mg/litre and the presumption was that the rain water had washed the lead into the river. There is a particularly great species variation amongst fish in their ability to tolerate lead. Goldfish seem to be resistant to its effects (Jones, 1938) probably because of their abundant gill secretion which washes away the film of coagulated mucus from the body and especially the gills, which would otherwise result in fatal anoxia (Ellis, 1937). On the other hand, concentrations of 0·1 mg/litre and upwards are fatal to minnows (Jones, 1938) and it is interesting that this species could not survive in some Glasgow tap water which averages 0·16 mg/litre (Ministry of Agriculture, 1972).

The presence of calcium in the water decreases the toxic effect of lead to fish (Jones, 1938), which is interesting in view of the effect calcium has in animals of decreasing absorption from the gut. Some marine animals show a remarkable facility for concentrating lead from their surroundings. Shell-fish, and in particular, oysters, are noteworthy in this respect (Pringle *et al.*, 1968).

Zoo animals are not exempt from lead poisoning and there have been cases of primates developing the disease after chewing the paint on the bars or woodwork of their cages, or from eating paint which was in the vicinity (Fisher, 1954; Hausman *et al.*, 1961, Sauer *et al.*, 1970). An outbreak of the disease in fruit bats was also linked to their chewing cage-bars painted with lead paint (Zook *et al.*, 1970).

An outbreak of lead poisoning amongst animals in the Staten Island and Bronx zoos was attributed to atmospheric contamination. Samples of vegetation within the confines of the zoos were found to contain up to 3,900 ppm of lead, and although there was lead in the paint, which had been supplied as being lead-free, the conclusion of the investigators was that most of the lead taken in by the animals resulted from atmospheric fall-out (Bazell, 1971).

2 Lead Metabolism

I. UPTAKE

Lead may be taken into the body by inhalation, ingestion or through the skin.

A. Uptake by the Lungs

The uptake of any inhaled particulate material is a function of its size and solubility. The size of the particle will determine the fraction which is deposited in the lung. Percentage deposition increases with particle size from a minimum of 25 per cent for particles approximately 0·5 μ in diameter to a maximum of almost 100 per cent for particles greater than 25 μ. Below 0·5 μ the deposition also increases so that for particles smaller than 0·1 μ the percentage deposited in the alveoli approaches 100 per cent (Fig. 16) (Hatch and Gross, 1964). Particles of hygroscopic material are deposited in the lungs in a higher percentage than non-hygroscopic because as they take up water from the moist air in the respiratory tract their size increases.

Deposition of inhaled particles will also vary with increased rates of inhalation. Minimum deposition occurs at a respiratory rate of about 15–20 l/min. At lower rates, there is an increased probability of particles settling out by gravity and diffusion of particles increases proportionately with the increase of transit time of the dust-laden air in and out of the lungs. At increased rates of respiration coarse particles are deposited in greater quantity because the force of inertial deposition rises with the increase in air velocity.

Particle size also determines the site in the respiratory system at which the inhaled material is deposited. In the nasal cavities almost all the particles greater than 10 μ are removed but removal is virtually zero at about 1 μ. This means that the percentage penetration of particles in

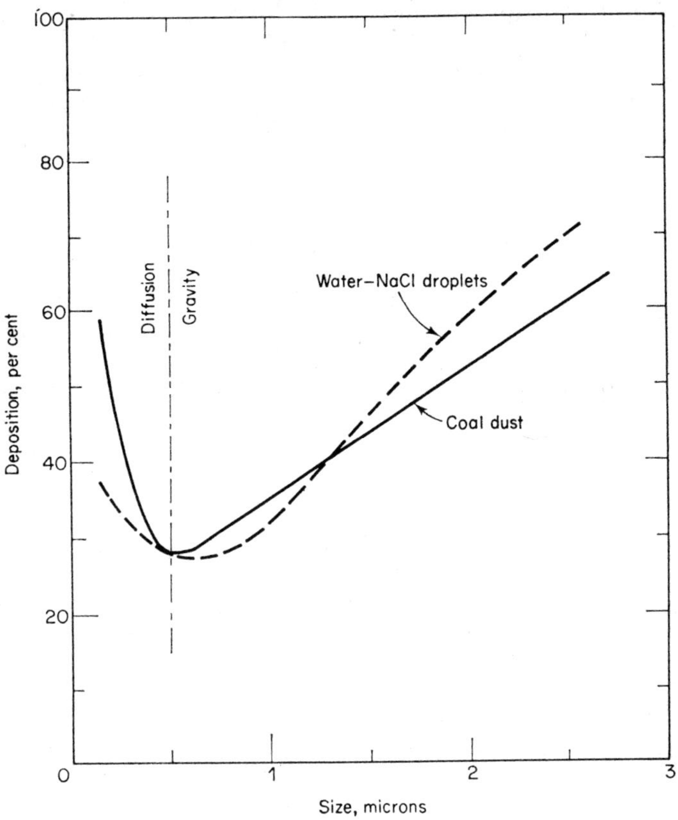

FIG. 16. Percentage of respiratory deposition in relation to particle size. Reproduced with permission from Dautrebande and Walkenhorst (1961).

the pulmonary air spaces rises from zero at 10 μ to a maximum for particles equal or greater than 1 μ. Removal of particles from the air increases as size decreases down to about 2 μ and falls to a minimum at about 0·5 μ. Below 0·5 μ the percentage removed increases as the force of precipitation by diffusion increases.

Clearance of particles from the lungs occurs when the inhaled material is sequestered by alveolar cells or removed via the lymphatic vessels to local lymph nodes. Alternatively, it may dissolve in the tissue fluids and pass into the blood. The rate of passage of an inhaled substance into the blood will depend on its particle size and solubility, since these parameters will determine the rate at which it will go into solution. As particle size decreases and solubility increases, so the proportion of material passing into the blood will increase with respect to the amount cleared from the lungs by sequestration or lymph drainage.

It has been demonstrated many times that these considerations apply equally to inhaled lead as to any other material. Kehoe (1961a, b, 1964a) found that the retention of lead sesquioxide particles in the lung ranged from 35 per cent when the mean particle diameter was 0·05 μ, up to 54 per cent for a diameter of 0·75 μ. When the mean diameter was approximately 1 μ, retention was 43 to 53 per cent. Values for the retention of inhaled lead of between 37 and 47 per cent, similar to those of Kehoe were found by Mehani (1966) but unfortunately the particle size was not determined. In a study using ^{212}Pb, Hursh and Mercer (1970) found the percentage of lead deposited after inhalation in 4 subjects varied from 27 to 62 per cent and was dependent on particle size (Table 18).

Table 18

Deposition of ^{212}Pb in the lungs and its relation to particle size

Subject	% of inhaled lead retained	Particle size, μ[a]
A	38	0·20
B	27	0·23
C	50	0·025
D	62	<0·02

[a] Mean aerodynamic diameter.
From Hursh and Mercer (1970)

Tetra-ethyl lead vapour is absorbed through the pulmonary epithelium with great facility (Kehoe, 1925, 1927). Mortensen (1942) studied the uptake of tetra-ethyl lead from the lungs in rats using radium-D as a marker. He found that the amount absorbed was in proportion to the concentration of vapour in the inhaled air, although it fell off at high concentrations (Table 19). He calculated that in a saturated atmosphere containing 7·0 mg of lead tetra-ethyl per litre, 16 per cent of the material reaching the pulmonary epithelium is absorbed. This figure rises to 23 per cent at one-hundredth saturation.

The clearance of lead from the lungs has been studied using lead radio-isotopes. The values for the half-life of lead in the lungs, reported by

Table 19

Effect of concentration on absorption of tetra-ethyl lead in rats

Vapour conc. mg/litre	Mean TEL absorbed mg/kg	Ratio of amount absorbed to conc.
0·07	0·24	3·4
0·15	0·53	3·5
0·51	1·52	3·0
1·03	3·19	3·1
2·50	6·34	2·5
7·00	16·90	2·4

From Mortensen (1942)

Table 20

Clearance of ^{212}Pb from the lungs

Author	Half-life (hr)
Jacobi (1964)	8
Hursh *et al.* (1969)	6·5
Booker *et al.* (1969)	approx. 10
Hursh and Mercer (1970)	10·5–11·5

different authors, have been in good agreement and are shown in Table 20. In general these results confirm Kehoe's (1961b) conclusion that the absorption of sub-micron particles from the lung would be complete within 24 hr.

Table 21 lists the solubility of some of the more common lead compounds whilst Table 22 shows their relative toxicity. The correlation between toxicity and aqueous solubility is not absolute, but it is the solubility of the lead compounds in tissue fluids which is of prime importance in determining their passage into the blood. The solubility of some lead compounds in pleural fluid and blood serum is shown in Table 23. It will be seen that the values are markedly different from those shown for the same compounds in Table 22, all being significantly more soluble in tissue fluids than in water.

Table 21

Solubility of some common lead compounds

Compound	Formula	Molecular weight	Solubility, mg/100 ml water at 20°C[a]
Titanate	$PbTiO_3$	303·09	Insoluble
Silicate	$PbSiO_3$	283·27	Insoluble
Red oxide (minium)	Pb_3O_4	685·57	Insoluble
Dioxide	PbO_2	239·19	Insoluble
Chromate	$PbCrO_4$	323·18	0·058^{25}
Carbonate (cerussite)	$PbCO_3$	267·20	1·10
Mono-oxide (litharge)	PbO	223·19	17·0
Sulphate	$PbSO_4$	303·25	42·50^{25}
Sulphide (galena)	PbS	239·25	124·40
Hydroxide	$Pb(OH)_2$	464·39	155·0
Stearate	$Pb(C_{18}H_{35}O_2)_2$	774·15	500·0^{35}
Di-iodide	PbI_2	461·00	630·0
Fluoride	PbF_2	245·19	640·0
Mono-iodide	PbI	334·09	1000·0
Bromide	$PbBr_2$	367·01	8441·0
Chloride	$PbCl_2$	278·10	9900·0
Nitrate	$Pb(NO_3)_2$	331·20	37·65 × $10^{4°}$
Acetate	$Pb(C_2H_3O_2)_2$	325·28	44·3 × 10^4

[a] Superscript numbers by figures in the last column indicate temperature in °C where this differs from 20

The potential increase in the body burden of lead from inhalation has been given by Knelson *et al.* (1972) as

$$L \times V \times R \times D \times 10^{-3}\,\mu g/\text{day where}$$
$$L = \text{Air lead concentration } \mu g/m^3$$
$$V = \text{Pulmonary ventilation } m^3/\text{day}$$
$$R = \text{Fraction of inhaled lead retained}$$
$$D = \text{Duration of exposure in days.}$$

From this, they constructed a model describing lead uptake and excretion kinetics for persons exposed to atmospheric lead. This model provides useful data, to which reference is given again later, but it should be remembered that the values of R will vary according to the solubility and particle size of the particular lead compounds. In the model the authors have assumed a constant value of thirty-seven per cent.

Table 22

Relative toxicity of lead and its compounds

Order of toxicity	Method of introduction		
	Injection	Ingestion	Inhalation
Most toxic	Lead arsenate	Lead arsenate Lead carbonate Lead monoxide Lead sulphate	Lead carbonate Lead monoxide
Of similar but a lower degree of toxicity	Metallic lead Lead carbonate Lead chromate Lead monoxide Red lead Lead dioxide Lead phosphate Lead sulphate Lead sulphide	Metallic lead Lead chromate Red lead Lead dioxide Lead phosphate Lead sulphide	Metallic lead Lead arsenate Lead chromate Red lead Lead dioxide Lead phosphate Lead silicate Lead sulphide

From Fairhall and Sayers (1940)

Table 23

Solubility of some lead compounds in human pleural fluid and blood serum

Compound	Solubility mg/litre	Temp °C
Titanate (purified)	0·287	36
Titanate (commercial)	0·477	33
Chromate	1·14	30–33
Carbonate	9·62	30
	10·64	36

From Harrold (1949)

B. Gastrointestinal Absorption

It is probable that under normal conditions not more than five to ten per cent of ingested lead is absorbed from the gut (Kehoe *et al.*, 1933a,b,c, 1940a, 1943; Kehoe, 1961a, 1964a). In exceptional cases figures in excess of this have been quoted, for example 16 per cent in one subject (Hursh and Suomela, 1968) and Imamura has quoted a figure of up to 40 per cent (Imamura, 1957). In man, the generally accepted quotient of intestinal absorption is 0·08 in adults although this average figure conceals wide individual variations. In children this quotient is much greater, perhaps as high as 0·25 or 0·50 (Karhausen, 1972; Alexander *et al.*, 1972). Table 24 shows the data from one of the

Table 24

Lead input and output during a two year period of oral administration in a normal subject

	mgm	% of total
Ingested:		
In drinking water	12·00	0·8
In food and beverages	120·48	8·5
Administered in solution	1286·85	90·7
TOTAL	1419·33	100·0
Excreted:		
In faeces	1236·19	87·1
In urine	73·07	5·1
TOTAL	1309·26	92·2
Retained	110·07	7·8

From Kehoe *et al.* (1943)

experiments conducted with normal subjects performed by Kehoe and his colleagues (1943), and is typical.

In animals, the amount of lead absorbed from the gut appears to be less than in man. Sheep and rabbits, for example, take up less than 1·5 per cent of administered lead over a range of 2–108 mgPb/day (Blaxter, 1950). Nor does the form in which lead is administered appear to affect its absorption. Calves, poisoned with a series of lead salts, showed little difference in uptake when the lead was given as the acetate, phosphate, oxide or carbonate, or even as dried paint flakes. Only galena and metallic lead appeared to be absorbed poorly (Allcroft. 1950). Karhausen (1972) however, states that galena is readily absorbed from the gut in the presence of gastric acid secretions. According to this author, the lead sulphide is converted to lead chloride which may then be absorbed. Any chloride remaining is converted back into lead sulphide in the colon.

Most of the lead which is taken into the alimentary tract is a contaminant of food or drink, but as much as 40 per cent of inhaled lead of large diameter which is trapped in the upper respiratory tract may be swallowed (Kehoe, 1961a).

In general, uptake of lead from the gut is less complete than it is from the lungs. Horiuchi (1965) for example, found that whereas 31·8 per cent of inhaled lead (as RaD) was absorbed it was true for only 5·3 per cent of an oral dose. The mechanism whereby lead is transported across the gut mucosa has not been worked out, but a number of factors are known to influence lead uptake, in particular the amount of calcium and phosphate in the diet. Shields and Mitchell (1941) showed that the concentration of lead in the soft tissues was increased by lowering the amounts of calcium and phosphate in the diet, either separately or together; an effect more recently confirmed by Six and Goyer (1970). These authors found that rats receiving lead at 200 ppm in their drinking water, but also on a low calcium diet, had blood lead concentrations approximately four times higher than rats exposed to the same lead concentration but on a normal calcium intake. Femur concentration of lead was also raised in the group on low calcium, by a factor of three compared with the control group. The same phenomenon has also been demonstrated in man by Crawford and Crawford (1969). In a series of autopsies the rib lead concentration was significantly higher in those patients who had lived in soft-water as opposed to hard-water districts (93 ppm compared with 54 ppm, $p < 0{\cdot}001$). This effect seems specific for gastrointestinal absorption since Lederer and Bing (1940) demonstrated that low calcium levels did not increase the uptake of lead administered intraperitoneally.

It has been postulated that calcium reduces lead absorption from the gut by competing for binding sites on mucosal cells, the effect being an example of competitive inhibition. An active transport system may be involved, however, perhaps governed in part by the influence of vitamin D. The presence of vitamin D in the diet increased the concentration of lead in the blood (Sobel *et al.*, 1940; Sobel and Burger, 1955), and in the femur (Sobel *et al.*, 1938). This effect has also been noted in children (Rapoport and Rubin, 1941), and might explain why outbreaks of lead poisoning amongst children are greatest in the summer months (Chisholm and Harrison, 1956). If there is an active transport system, then it functions differently during early life, since absorption of lead from the gut in neonates is very high (Kostial *et al.*, 1971a, b). For example, neonatal rats absorb about 60 per cent of the lead in their mothers' milk (Kostial *et al.*, 1971b). Growing animals absorb more from the gut than adults (Shields *et al.*, 1938) but this effect is lessened in the presence of adequate dietary calcium (Kostial *et al.*, 1971c).

It has also been postulated that during maturation the gut mucosal cells develop the ability to reject a number of multivalent cations, including lead, strontium and iron, which the immature gut absorbs avidly (Forbes and Reina, 1972).

An alternative hypothesis is that the presence of high concentrations of phosphate in the diet leads to the formation of insoluble lead phosphate (Kostial *et al.*, 1971b). Kostial and his colleagues (1969, 1971b) have also shown that the addition of alginates to the diet of neonatal rats decreases the absorption of lead from milk but this has not been confirmed by other workers (Harrison *et al.*, 1969; Carr *et al.*, 1969).

C. Absorption Through the Skin

Absorption through the skin is of importance only in the case of organic compounds of lead, particularly the lead alkyls and lead naphthenates (Pettinati *et al.*, 1959; Rassetti *et al.*, 1961). Soon after lead tetra-ethyl was introduced into commercial use, Eldridge (1924) reported that it was absorbed through the skin with great facility in both dogs and guinea-pigs. The presence of gasoline has been said to delay the penetration of tetra-ethyl lead through the skin (Kehoe and Thamann, 1931), although it has no effect on its uptake by the lungs (Mortensen ,1942).

The rate of absorption of tetra-ethyl lead and inorganic compounds through the skin was studied by Lang and Kunze (1948). They applied solutions of lead acetate, orthoarsenate, oleate and tetra-ethyl lead to the bare skin of a number of rats and measured the amount of lead in the kidney as an index of absorption. In all cases, the amount of lead in the kidney was greater than in controls, but only when tetra-ethyl lead had been applied did the difference assume any magnitude (Table 25). If the skin was traumatized before the lead solutions were applied, it was found that there was a three- or four-fold increase in renal lead concentration.

Table 25

Cutaneous absorption of lead compounds

Compound	Quantity applied mg/g	Lead conc. in kidneys wet wt.	Control
Arsenate	102	0·85	0·55
Oleate	148	1·30	0·59
Acetate	77	1·80	0·82
Tetra-ethyl	106	64·20	

From Lang and Kunze (1948)

II. FATE OF ABSORBED LEAD

A. Uptake by the Blood

The transfer of lead from the external to the internal environment is poorly understood but there is a considerable body of data concerning its transport in the blood.

In the blood, lead is present bound to the red cell or to the plasma proteins, and a small amount is in a free ionized form. Most of the lead in the blood, probably in excess of ninety-five per cent of the circulating total, is bound to the red cell (Clarkson and Kench, 1958), but this figure is dose-dependant. In dogs, 97 to 99 per cent of an injected dose calculated to give a concentration of 1 mg per cent is bound to the red cells. With higher doses (up to 100 mg per cent), saturation is reached and only 35 per cent of the dose becomes bound to the cell. The lead in the blood is in dynamic equilibrium between the plasma and the red cells so that lead is given up from the cells as the plasma concentration falls (Mortensen and Kellogg, 1944). The capacity of the red cells to hold lead may show individual variation from one person to another (Müller, 1950).

The speed of uptake by the cells is very rapid and shows similar characteristics both *in vivo* and *in vitro* (Fig. 17). Shortly after absorption, a substantial percentage of lead appears bound to the red cell. Estimates of the actual percentage vary, but it is evidently dose-dependant (Schubert and White, 1952; Hevesy and Nylin, 1953; Stover, 1959; Hursh and Suomela, 1968; Booker *et al.*, 1969; Hursh and Mercer, 1970).

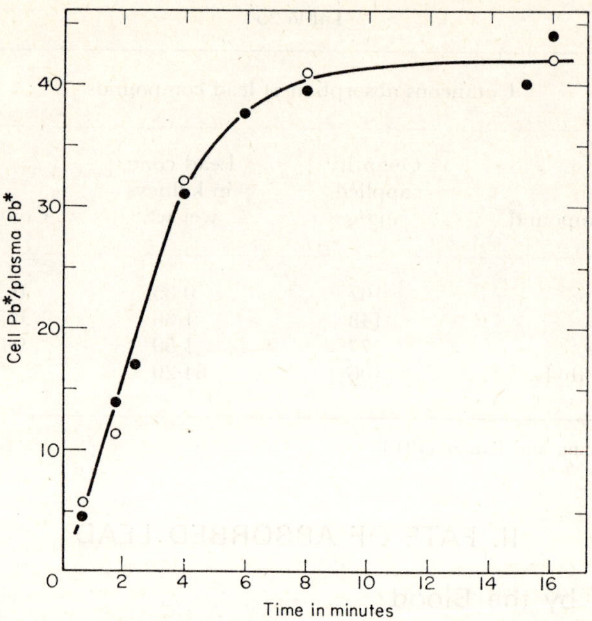

FIG. 17. The transfer of labelled lead from the plasma to the cells at body temperature. Solid circles: *in vivo*; open circles: *in vitro*. Reproduced with permission from Mortensen and Kellogg (1944).

The rate of lead uptake by the red cells from the plasma is also temperature-dependant (Fig. 18). Mortensen and Kellogg (1944) suggested that their data showed that the uptake of lead by the erythrocytes was a first order reaction until about 85 per cent completed with a specific rate of 0·058 and 0·60/min at 0° and 20°C respectively. Substitution of this datum into the Arrhenius equation gave a value of 21,000 calories/mole for the energy of activation. Utilizing this datum for a temperature of 38°C they estimated that 50 per cent of a dose of lead in a concentration of 0·1 mg per cent should be taken up in 0·17 minutes and 85 per cent in 0·5 minutes. Clarkson and Kench (1958), however, considered the data from their experiments best fitted a second order reaction (Fig. 19) and that redrawing Mortensen and Kellogg's data for second-order kinetics gave excellent linearity. They confirmed that the uptake from the plasma was markedly influenced by temperature and from the data in Fig. 19 showed that the ratio of the velocities of uptake at 10° and 20°C was given by the equation:

$$k20°/k10° = 5{\cdot}61 \times 10^4/2{\cdot}16 \times 10^4/\text{minute},$$

thus $Q_{10} = 2{\cdot}8$

and energy of activation = 15,800 cal/mole.

The energy of activation derived from this experiment is typical of chemisorption rather than physical absorption. The sites of binding to the red cell are found on the cell membrane which has a particular affinity for lead (Watanabe and Yana, 1953). The lead is probably bound to the lipids and lipoproteins in the cell membrane (Jung, 1947; Teisinger *et al.*, 1958). Lipid-free stroma does not bind lead effectively (Vincent, 1958) and cells which have passed through alumina are insensitive to the effects of lead (Passow *et al.*, 1961). Since alumina removes cholesterol, phospholipids and lipoproteins from red blood cells (Lovelock, 1955), it seems

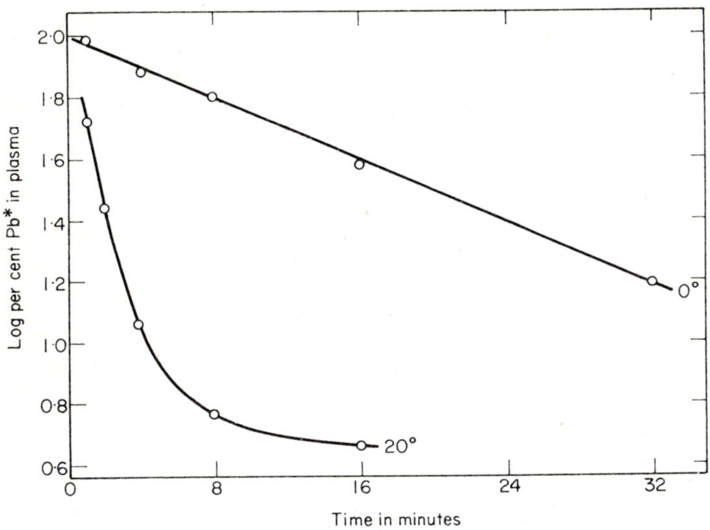

Fig. 18. The rate of disappearance of labelled lead from the plasma of whole blood at 0° and 20°C. Reproduced with permission from Mortensen and Kellogg (1944).

reasonable to suppose that these are the agents responsible for binding lead to the membrane. In the case of tetra-ethyl lead the proportion of lipid-bound lead is higher than for inorganic compounds (Beattie *et al.*, 1972c).

It is probable that lead is bound to the red cell as a peptized lead phosphate sol (Clarkson and Kench, 1958) which then aggregates to form a mosaic on the inner surface of the membrane (Jung, 1956), although other possibilities have been put forward by earlier workers. Aub *et al.* (1925) considered lead to be present as a colloidal di-lead phosphate whereas Maxwell and Bischoff (1929a, b) thought it was in the form of the diphosphoglycerate. Another suggestion was that the lead in the blood formed mixed salts with calcium and chloride (Jowett, 1932).

Reddi (1953) has indicated that there may be two components responsible for lead uptake on the red cell, one consisting of protein and the other non-protein, probably a phenolic compound.

Like other heavy metals, lead has an affinity towards sulphydryl (-SH) groups particularly di-thiol groups, and it is one of the most active of the heavy metals in this respect. (The order of activity is Hg > Ag > Pb > Cd > Zn > Ca > Mg). It has been suggested that in the presence

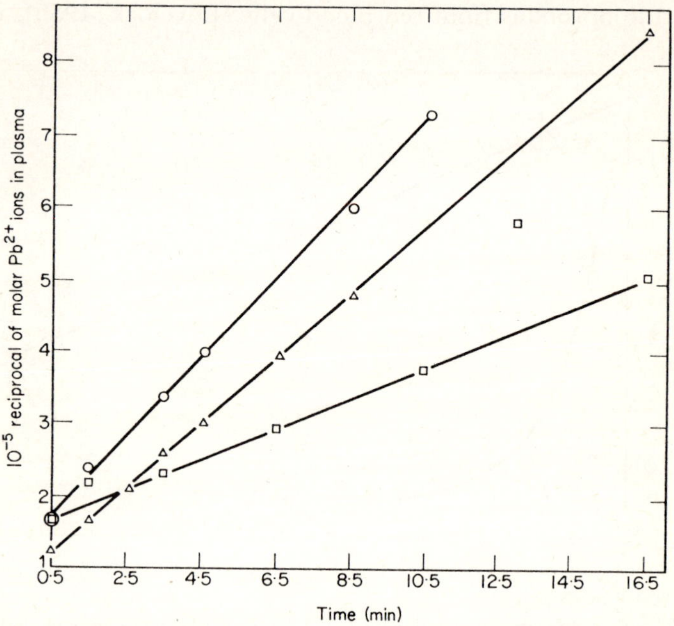

FIG. 19. Uptake of lead by human erythrocytes in oxalated whole blood at 20° (△) and in whole heparinized blood at 10° (□) and 20° (○). Results are plotted as a test for second-order kinetics with respect to lead. Reproduced with permission from Clarkson and Kench (1958).

of lead a series of reactions takes place on the membrane (Passow and Tillman, 1956). First, an S—S bridge breaks open to give a S—Pb complex, after which a S—Pb—S complex is slowly formed.

In the plasma, lead is bound to the plasma proteins (Teisinger, 1935; Tanford, 1950; Cund and Murray, 1954). Numerous sites exist for binding in the plasma, for in common with other heavy metals, lead may complex with ligands which contain S, N, or O as electron donors, for example —OH, —COOH, —PO_3H_2, —SH, —NH_2, -imidazole. It readily binds to amino acids although less avidly than to —SH groups.

Here the order of activity is Hg > Cu > Ni > Pb > Zn > Co > Cd > Mn > Ca > Ba (Passow *et al.*, 1961).

Lead disappears from the blood at a rate which follows first-order reaction kinetics and may be the sum of as many as three exponential functions (Castellino and Aloj, 1964; Fig. 20). The rate of disappearance from the blood of a single large dose of lead injected intravenously is shown in Fig. 21 (Hopkins, 1970). Stover (1959) postulated from her

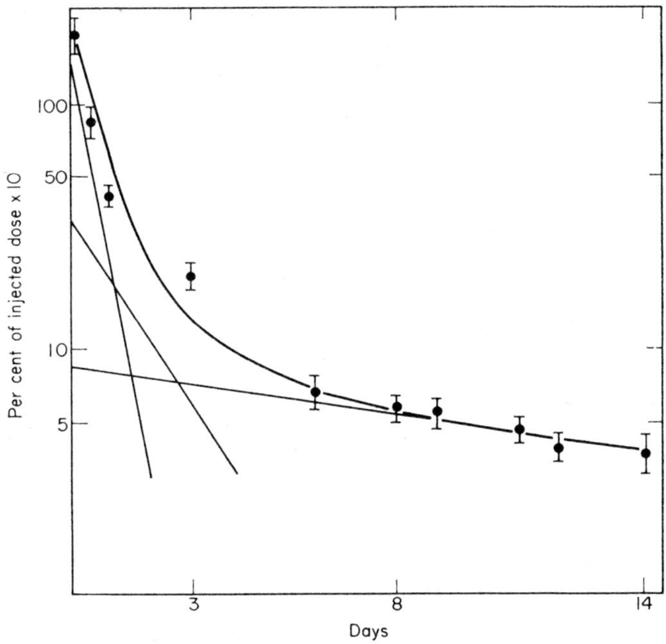

FIG. 20. Variation with time of ^{210}Pb content of whole blood. Reproduced with permission from Castellino and Aloj (1964).

experiments that lead rapidly transferred to the extravascular space from the plasma but there was a partial return of lead from the extravascular space as the plasma level declined. There is a dynamic equilibrium between red cell and plasma lead on the one hand and extracellular and intracellular lead on the other (Fig. 22). It is likely to be the ionic fraction of the plasma lead which is transferable to other body compartments.

Release of lead from the red cells may be relatively slow, and Hursch and Soumela have advanced the theory that it may only happen on the death of the red cell. Many of the data which they use to verify this suggestion are speculative, however, and such a concept is difficult to reconcile with a system in dynamic equilibrium. Barltrop's (1969) finding

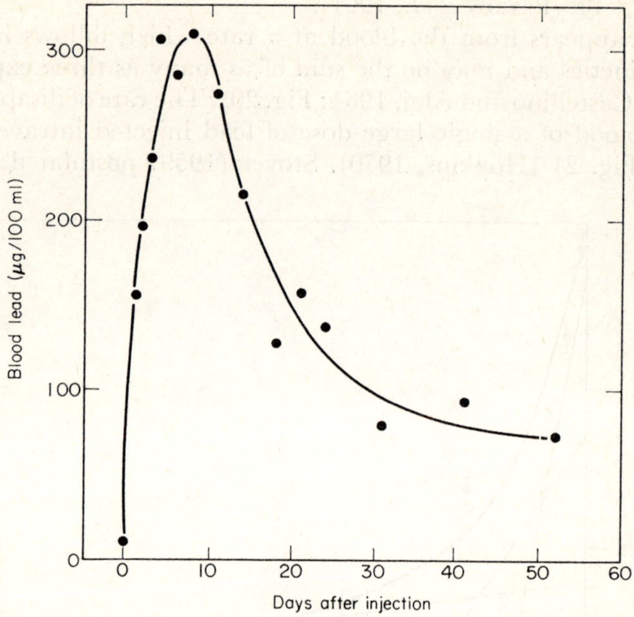

FIG. 21. The changes in the blood lead concentration of a baboon after a single injection of 1,000 mg of lead carbonate. Reproduced with permission from Hopkins (1970).

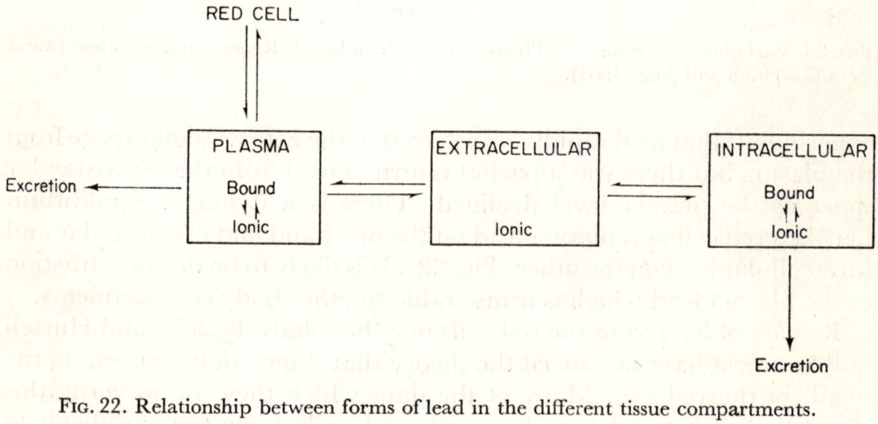

FIG. 22. Relationship between forms of lead in the different tissue compartments.

that the biological half-life of lead in rabbit erythrocytes is about 2·5 days also mitigates strongly against this theory.

B. Uptake of Lead by Soft Tissues

Lead diffuses from the plasma into the extravascular space and then enters the cells. The kinetics of removal of lead from the soft tissues closely resemble those of its removal from the blood (Figs 23–26). The exchange

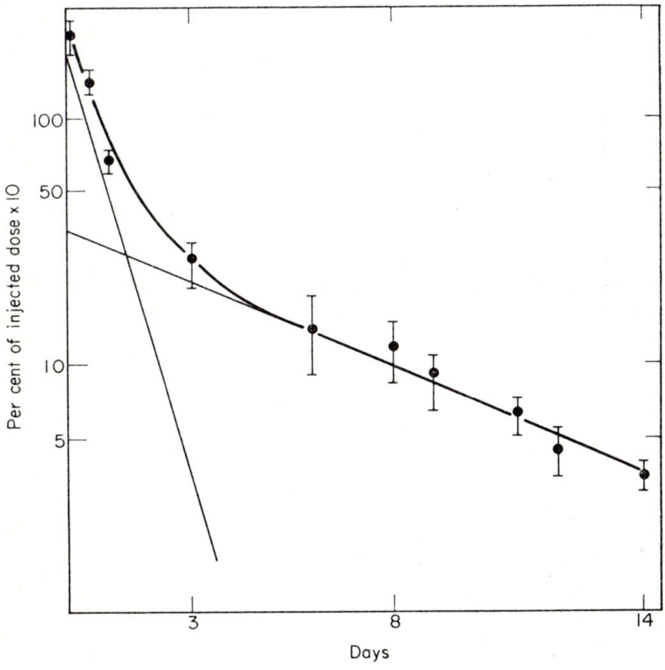

FIG. 23. Variation with time of ^{210}Pb content of the liver. Reproduced with permission from Castellino and Aloj (1964).

rates for muscle and skin, however, are slower than those of other soft tissues (Bolanowska *et al.*, 1964). Lead appears in the cells of the liver and kidney within an hour of injection (Castellino and Aloj, 1969), and appears to be particularly strongly bound to the mitochondria (Fig. 27). Repeated washing fails to remove all the lead from mitochondria and this strong affinity is of particular relevance when the pathological effects of lead come to be considered (Ch. 3).

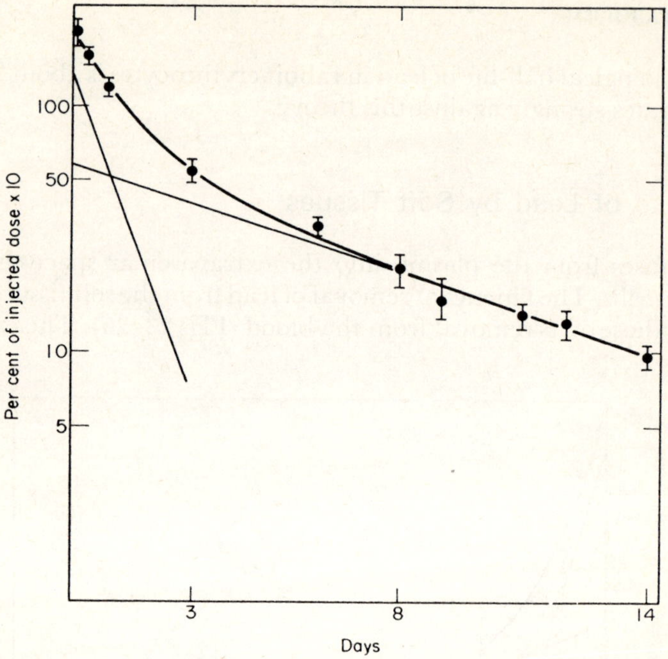

FIG. 24. Variation with time of ^{210}Pb content of the kidney. Reproduced with permission from Castellino and Aloj (1964).

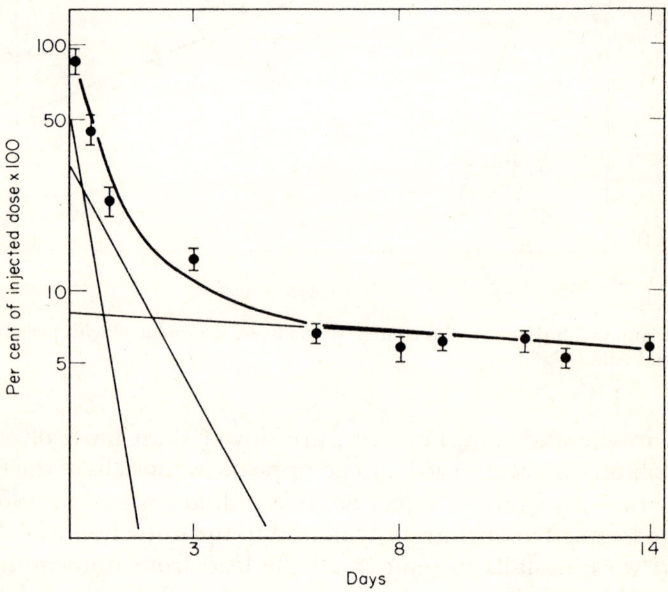

FIG. 25. Variation with time of ^{210}Pb content of the lung. Reproduced with permission from Castellino and Aloj (1964).

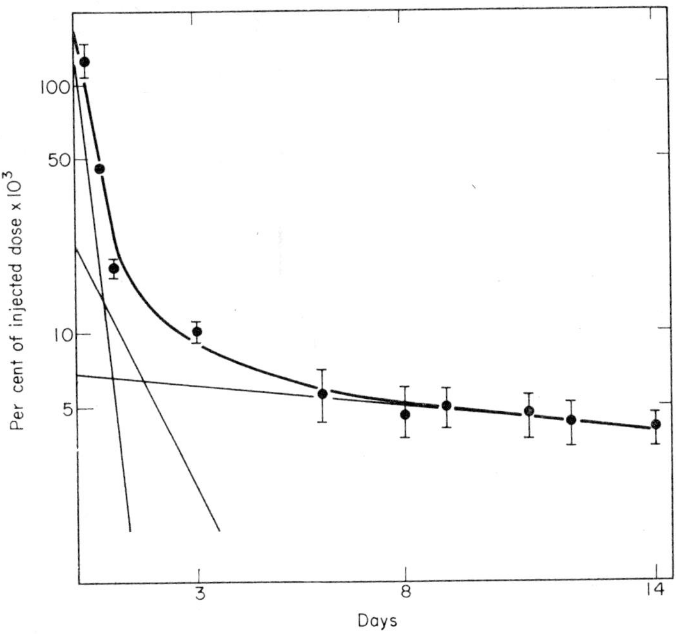

FIG. 26. Variation with time of ^{210}Pb content of heart. Reproduced with permission from Casellino and Aloj (1964).

C. Uptake by Bone

In the stable state about 90 per cent or more of the total body lead is stored in the skeleton and the metal has been graphically described as a bone-seeker (Hammond, 1969). In particular, it seeks out areas of active bone formation (Behrens and Baumann, 1933–1934). Bone mineral consists of two calcium phosphate pools which are chemically and physically distinct. The first is a crystalline phase consisting of apatite crystals similar to hydroxyapatite and the second is an amorphous non-crystalline phase composed predominately of calcium and phosphate (Posner, 1969). Bone apatite crystals are similar to but not identical with hydroxyapatite and the size and shape of the crystals varies with bone age and with diet. Lead, like strontium, can replace calcium in the calcium position of the crystal. The crystalline structure of bone gives a very large interface for reactions to take place which may be as much as 180 m^2/g (Eanes and Posner, 1967), and bone may be considered as a dynamic structure although only about 0·65 per cent of bone calcium is exchangeable (Rowland, 1966).

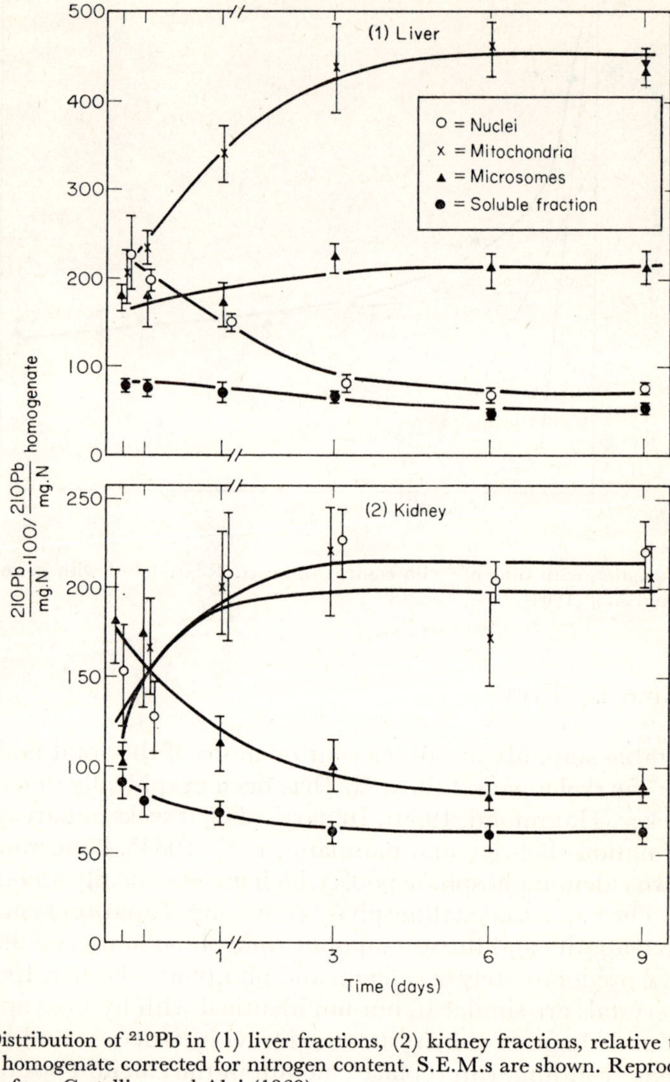

FIG. 27. Distribution of ^{210}Pb in (1) liver fractions, (2) kidney fractions, relative to ^{210}Pb in the whole homogenate corrected for nitrogen content. S.E.M.s are shown. Reproduced with permission from Castellino and Aloj (1969).

Early investigators demonstrated that pulverized bone took up lead in proportion to the amount of calcium lost, suggesting simple ionic exchange (Aub *et al.*, 1926). More recent work using X-ray diffraction has indicated that the lead assumes a position within the bone crystal either by displacing other cations or by occupying lattice interstices (McDonald *et al.*, 1951), but this does not exclude the possibility that the lead may also be bound to organic components of the bone or deposited as a discrete crystal of an insoluble compound. At very low concentrations, lead is an effective nucleating agent for inducing formation of calcium phosphate crystals and this mechanism may be important in trapping lead at the surface of the bone crystal (Fleisch *et al.*, 1965). It is

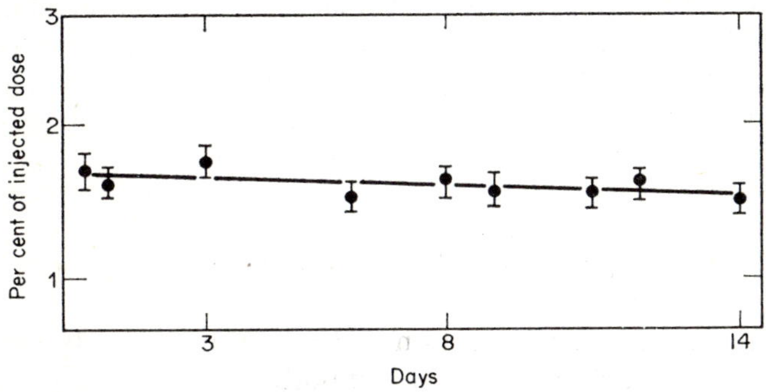

FIG. 28. Variation with time of ^{210}Pb content of bone. Reproduced with permission from Castellino and Aloj (1964).

probable that lead is first deposited in the trabeculae and then migrates to the cortical bone (McLean *et al.*, 1954). The importance of lead in soft-tissue calcification may be in its effect as a nucleating agent in addition to its ability to attract calcium to sites of irritation (Selye *et al.*, 1964a, b, c; Selye and Somogyi, 1968).

The reasons why lead and calcium seem interchangeable in bone are not clear. Aub and his colleagues picturesquely described lead as flowing in the calcium stream in the body and contended that the two elements shared a common metabolism. This appeared to be substantiated by the finding that parathormone enhanced the mobilization of both lead and calcium in man (Hunter and Aub, 1926–1927), although this was not the case in dogs, even when the serum calcium was high, or the amount of calcium in the diet was varied (Calhoun *et al.*, 1954).

Although it is often assumed that lead in bone is in a fixed and non-diffusible form it is removed at a very slow and constant rate (Fig. 28). The biological half-time for the loss of radio-lead from the human skeleton is

670 to 840 days (Black, 1962). There is some ill-defined evidence that under certain circumstances lead may be released more rapidly from the bone. Factors which have been incriminated include acute or chronic infections, disturbances of acid/base balance, fever, fractures and excessive alcohol intake (Cantarow and Trumper, 1944; Schwartz, 1951; Byers and Maloof, 1954; King and Thompson, 1961). Malignant invasion of the medullary cavities releases sufficient lead to raise the blood-lead concentrations of affected patients above the mean of both normal controls and of patients with other diseases, including malignant disease without secondary spread to the bone (Brown, 1946). If the patient has had considerable exposure in the past, enough lead may be released to produce signs of clinical poisoning and Brown and Tompsett (1945) report such a case in a compositor who had leukaemic hyperplasia of the bone marrow. Although, in general, objective evidence to support these claims is lacking, it is reasonable to suppose that if lead and calcium are metabolized similarly in bone, then factors which tend to release one will also release the other.

III. EXCRETION OF LEAD

The principal routes of elimination of lead from the body are via the faeces and the urine. Faecal excretion of both inorganic and organic lead is greater than urinary excretion (Kehoe, 1925), and for inorganic lead, the ratio of lead content is approximately 100:1 (Kehoe, 1964a). Perceptible sweat contains lead in a concentration about equal to that of the urine. Lead can be excreted in milk but the concentrations are very small (Table 26).

Table 26

Lead content of human milk

Sample	Volume, ml	Total lead content μg	Concentration μg/litre
1	2031	50	24·6
2	1936	100	51·6
3	2806	90	32·1
4	1280	40	31·3
5	2858	nil	

From Kehoe *et al.* (1933d)

Most of the lead in the faeces represents ingested lead which has passed unabsorbed through the gut. The classical studies of Kehoe's group indicate that not more than 10 per cent of ingested lead is absorbed, although this is an average figure and there is wide individual variation. This lead is, properly speaking, not excreted lead since it has not been metabolized through the body, and in the discussion which follows, only absorbed lead is considered. Estimates of the relative amounts of lead excreted in the faeces and the urine range from one to five (di Ferrante and Bourdeau, 1972) but in general, the gut is considered as the major route of lead excretion.

A. Excretion of Lead Through the Gut

Lead excreted in the faeces may come theoretically from one of two sources, the bile and pancreatic fluid, or the intestinal wall. Massione (1941) and Witschi (1964) both suggested that lead passed into the gut lumen bound to seralbumin and was there proteolysed to release free lead. Most observations, however, favour the view that lead excreted in the faeces derives predominantly from the bile. Blaxter and Cowie (1946) demonstrated this in the sheep. After administration of lead acetate, 7·5 per cent of the dose was excreted in 6 days of which 81 per cent was in the bile, and radio-lead studies have amply confirmed this (Castellino *et al.*, 1965, 1966; Cikrt, 1972) (Fig. 29). Cikrt's experiments, however, show that the cells of the gut wall do contain lead (Fig. 30) and may contribute to the overall excretion in small measure.

B. Through the Kidney

The renal excretion of a substance may be studied by measuring its clearance. This is defined from the formula

$$C = \frac{UV}{P} \text{ where } C = \text{clearance in ml/min}$$

$$U = \text{urine concentration mg \%}$$

$$V = \text{urine volume/min}$$

$$P = \text{plasma concentration mg \%}$$

and represents the amount of the substance removed from the plasma in unit time.

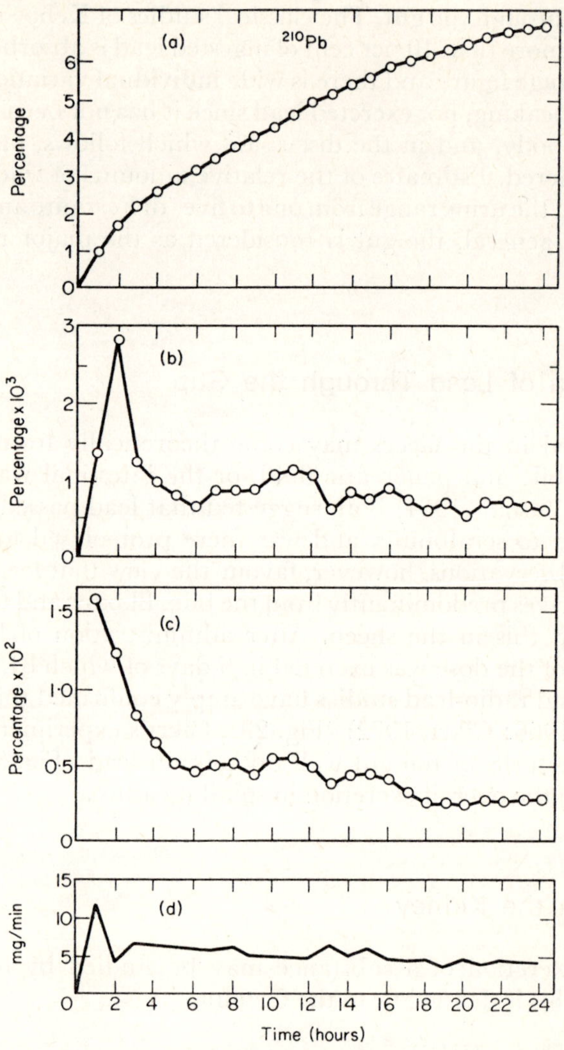

FIG. 29. A. Cumulative biliary excretion of ^{210}Pb as a percentage of the administered dose. B. Percentage of excreted ^{210}Pb/mg of bile. C. Excretion of ^{210}Pb as a percentage of the administered dose/min. D. Bile flow (mg/min). Open circles: the bile samples of five rats were pooled and measured as single samples. Reproduced with permission from Cikrt (1972).

The difficulty in determining lead clearance has been in the accurate measurement of the plasma concentration.

Pinto *et al.* (1941), made an estimate of lead clearance utilizing whole blood lead concentration and obtained a mean of 0·284 (±0·103) ml/min. Since they were using whole blood as opposed to plasma concentration, however, this figure is likely to be a gross underestimate of the clearance.

Whether the renal tubule takes an active part in lead excretion is open to doubt. Vostál (1963, 1966) investigated lead excretion in man and dogs and found that at low blood lead levels the lead was eliminated

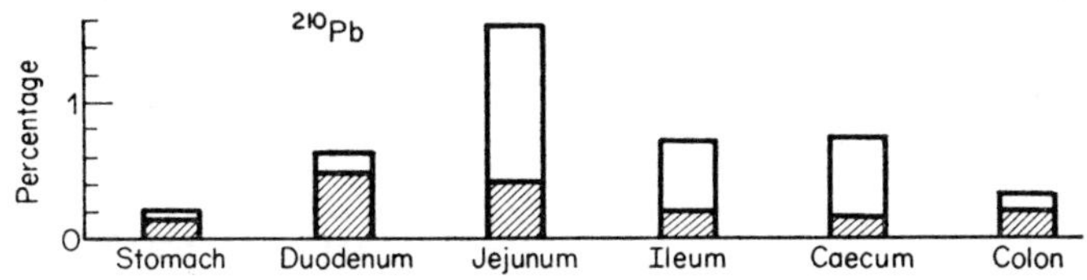

FIG. 30. Percentage of total dose of ^{210}Pb in the wall (hatched column) and the lumen (open column) of individual segments of the gastro-intestinal tract 24 hr after administration. Reproduced with permission from Cikrt (1972).

entirely by glomerular filtration as judged by the ratio of lead to creatinine clearance. With a sudden increase in blood lead concentration, brought about by an intravenous injection, a change was observed in the relationship between glomerular filtration rate and the amount of lead excreted. There was some evidence that the renal tubule was reabsorbing a constant amount of the filtered lead. This effect was pH-dependent. At low pH the amount of reabsorbed lead increased, but decreased, or entirely disappeared, if the pH was high. More recently it has been found that the renal tubule cell transports lead into the urine (Vostál and Heller, 1968) (Fig. 31), perhaps because of the presence of lead-binding ligands in the tubular cell. If intracellular ligands bind lead diffusing in from the extracellular fluid then the concentration gradient between the cell and the extracellular fluid will fall, resulting in the diffusion of more lead into the cell (Fig. 32).

IV. SPECIAL METABOLISM OF LEAD ALKYLS

TEL is insoluble in water but soluble in ethanol and fat solvents and it is probable that it is the water-soluble compounds of decomposition which are toxic rather than the parent compound itself (Buck and Kumro, 1930; Machle, 1935; Cremer, 1959). The contrary view has been forwarded by Kehoe (1925) and Cassells and Dodds (1946) who stated that the toxicity of TEL is a function of the lead content and that its fat-solvent properties determine its peculiar toxic features but the weight of opinion is against them.

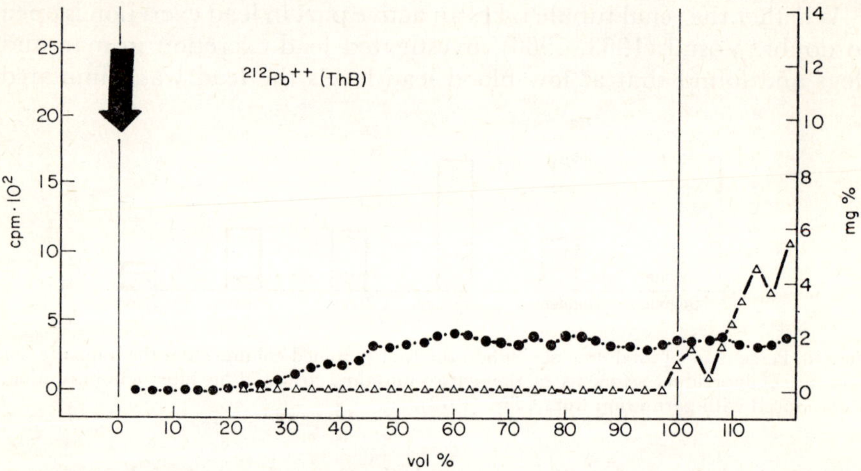

FIG. 31. Pattern of excretion of ^{212}Pb (●) and inulin (△) after an injection of 100 μCi ^{212}Pb at time indicated by the arrow. The concentrations were determined in single drops of urine collected from the left ureter. Individual drops are expressed on the abscissa as a percentage of the total volume of urine excreted by the kidney in the time interval between injection and first appearance of detectable traces of inulin. Reproduced with permission from Vostál and Heller (1968).

Under laboratory conditions, TEL is degraded to inorganic lead via triethyl and diethyl intermediates (Calingaert *et al.*, 1948; Henderson and Snyder, 1961).

$$(CH_3CH_2)_4Pb \rightarrow (CH_3CH_2)_3Pb^+ \rightarrow (CH_3CH_2)_2Pb^{2+} \rightarrow Pb^{2+}$$

Conversion to triethyl lead takes place rapidly in the liver (Cremer, 1959), but there is controversy concerning the formation of diethyl lead *in vivo*. Bolanowska (1968) considers that TEL is metabolized simultaneously to triethyl lead and inorganic lead as shown below.

$$(CH_3CH_2)_4Pb \nearrow (CH_3CH_2)_3Pb \quad \searrow Pb^{2+}$$

The conversion to inorganic lead proceeds more slowly than the conversion to lead triethyl (Bolanowska, 1968). It is highly unlikely, however, that four ethyl groups would be removed synchronously and the concensus of opinion is that diethyl lead is formed in the body. There is evidence that tetramethyl and tetrapropyl lead compounds are metabolized to the trialkyl form, but this conversion proceeds much more

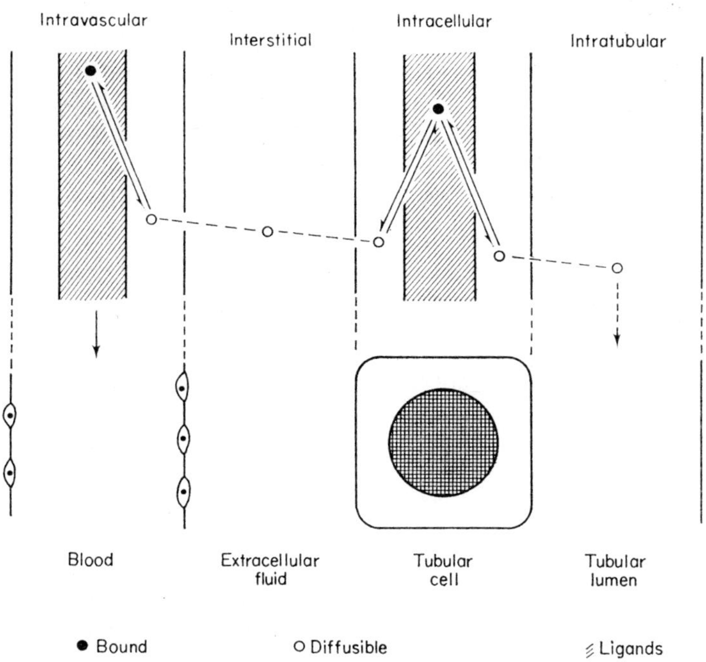

FIG. 32. Schematic drawing showing possible transport of diffusable fraction of lead following the concentration gradient across the renal compartments into the tubular fluid. Reproduced with permission from Vostál and Heller (1968).

slowly than the conversion of TEL to triethyl lead and may account for their being comparatively less toxic, although once formed, trimethyl lead compounds are as toxic as the triethyl (Cremer and Callaway, 1961).

It is important to remember that the distribution of organo-lead compounds differs from inorganic lead. Organo-lead compounds have no special affinity for bone but a high affinity for lipid-containing tissues, especially those constituting the nervous system. The brain and liver are amongst the organs with the highest concentration of organic lead. On the other hand, in rats at least, the placental barrier appears to be more effective in preventing the transport of organo-lead compounds than inorganic lead (McClain and Becker, 1972).

V. THE BODY BURDEN OF LEAD

When Devergie and Hervy (1838) first suggested that lead was present in normal persons, they sparked off a controversy which was not finally resolved until the advent of methods sensitive enough to detect trace amounts of lead with reasonable reliability. Today it is not questioned that each individual has a body burden of lead.

The body burden of lead may be described as the cumulative difference between the amounts of lead absorbed and excreted

$$\mathrm{B} = \Sigma(A - E)$$

where B = body burden

A = amount absorbed

E = amount excreted.

The body burden of environmental pollutants has been described by Goldsmith (1964) as the level of the polluting substance in the organs, blood, plasma or other body fluids of an organism, which produces or is capable of producing, damage or significant interference with body functions, or those of the organ or tissue. This definition, however, best describes the toxic threshold, ignoring as it does levels at which no ill effects are noted.

Most foreign substances disappear from the body in accordance with first-order kinetics and disappearance is proportional to the amount present at any given time, so that

$$A_t = A_0 \mathrm{e}^{-kt} \tag{1}$$

where A_0 = amount in the body at zero time

A_t = amount in the body at time t

k = rate constant.

With continued administration, a material obeying first order rules will attain equilibrium in the body if it is administered at a constant rate. The accumulation may be described thus:

$$A_t = \frac{A}{k}(1 - e^{-kt}) \tag{2}$$

where A = amount assimilated in unit time t and other definitions are as in (1) above.

Bone seekers such as lead do not obey first-order kinetics. The retention of a single dose of lead cannot be described using conventional exponential functions, since the fraction available for excretion becomes progressively smaller because the bone acts as a trap. Body retention for bone seekers is best described by power functions of the form

$$R_t = At^{-n}$$

where R = fraction of original dose at time t,
n = a constant equal to the slope of a linear log–log plot of R against t,
A = a constant equal to the fraction of the assimilated dose at
t = 1 day (Sanders, 1960; Hammond, 1969).

Other mathematical models have been suggested by Stirling *et al.* (1964) and Rustagi (1964, 1965).

A. Lead in Blood

Estimates of the range of blood lead values found in the population have varied, as might be expected when samples are taken from groups with presumed differences in exposure. The most comprehensive study has been that of Goldwater and Hoover (1967) who determined blood lead levels from persons in sixteen different countries. Their results are shown in Table 27.

In general, urban means tend to be higher than rural means. The Yugoslavian rural mean is exceptional in being more than twice the urban mean, but large areas of the country are highly plumbiferous and this should be borne in mind when analysing the data. It is more difficult to explain the high mean found in the aborigines of New Guinea who live in a comparatively non-industrialized environment. Too much emphasis should not be placed on this single observation, however, for it is counter to the trend towards a general rural–urban gradient (see also Table 28) and awaits confirmation.

No sex differences were noted in this study although earlier Hofreuter *et al.* (1961) were able to show variations amongst the urban and rural dwellers in Los Angeles with respect both to sex and smoking habits (Table 28). Kehoe and his group (Kehoe *et al.*, 1940b) found blood lead

Table 27

Blood lead concentrations in sixteen countries

	Blood lead concentration μg/100 ml					
Country	Urban			Rural		
	n	mean	SD	n	mean	SD
Argentina	43	16	10	6	9	5
Chile	34	18	6	1	15	
Czechoslovakia	20	20	8			
Egypt	19	23	16	9	12	9
England	30	23	13			
Finland	17	28	10	29	24	14
Holland	58	15	9	2	10	0
Israel	46	16	6	13	18	5
Italy	26	13	10			
Japan	32	21	11	8	18	7
Peru	32	7	8			
Poland	32	12	6	44	13	7
Sweden	14	9	3	16	10	3
Yugoslavia	30	15	6	16	32	14
United States						
California	27	19	4	6	17	4
New York City	105	17	18			
Ohio	20	18	10	20	12	6
New Guinea				28	22	5

From Goldwater and Hoover (1967)

concentrations of the same order as Goldwater and Hoover in a group of thirty Americans and thirty Mexicans.

A more detailed study by Kubota *et al.* (1968) investigated blood lead levels amongst residents in different areas in America. The overall mean was not markedly different from those reported by the earlier investigators although the means from one city to another varied widely as did the individual values within each city.

Black children who are deficient in the enzyme glucose-6-phosphate dehydrogenase have a higher blood lead concentration than those in whom the enzyme is present. This effect is due entirely to an increased

Table 28

Blood lead concentrations to show variation in urban and rural dwellers. Sex variations and effect of smoking are also shown

Group	Mean blood lead concentration μg/100 gm	
	Urban	Rural
Male	21	16
Female	16	10
Smokers	21	17
Non-smokers	17	11

From Hofreuter *et al.* (1961)

binding to the red cell; the serum lead concentration is actually lower than in normal children. This mechanism is obscure (McIntyre and Angle, 1972).

From these data it may be concluded that blood lead concentrations greater than 50 μg/100 ml are unlikely to occur in persons with no more than the general environmental exposure to lead and that the range of typical values lies between 10–40 μg/100 ml.

B. Soft Tissue Lead

The most extensive studies of soft-tissue lead distribution have been made by Schroeder and Tipton and their colleagues (Schroeder and Balassa, 1961; Tipton and Cook, 1963; Tipton and Schaefer, 1964; Tipton *et al.*, 1965; Schroeder and Tipton, 1968) and a recent survey has confirmed these earlier data (Barry and Mossman, 1970).

The concentration of lead in soft tissues varies according to the geographical origin of the material (Table 29) but in general it is found that the aorta has the highest lead concentration, followed by the liver and kidney. Distribution of lead is equal in both the cortex and medulla of the kidney. The brain, heart and muscle all show consistently low values.

Lead is found in significant concentrations in young children, even in stillbirths, indicating considerable exposure *in utero* (Table 30). Concentrations of lead in the soft tissues tend to increase with age, in material

Table 29

Variation in human soft tissue lead concentration with geographical location

Place of origin	n	Aorta	Liver	Kidney	Pancreas	Lung	Testis	Heart	Brain	Spleen	Bone
		Mean lead concentration, ppm ash									
Nine American cities	150	140	130	98	49	47	12	5	5	27	43
San Francisco	27	220	160	54	65	38	20	10	5	44	
Switzerland	9	32	59	45	42	32	23	14	5	20	
Africa	54	71	64	36	24	28	29	5	5	21	
Middle East	37	140	70	62	34	42	32	24	14	40	26
Far East	74	91	97	62	39	43	35	19	10	33	30

From Schroeder and Tipton (1968)

Table 30

Tissue lead concentration in children and adolescents

Place of origin	n	Aorta	Liver	Kidney	Pancreas	Lung	Testis	Heart	Brain	Spleen	Bone
		Mean lead concentration, ppm ash									
America											
Stillborn	22	65	53	38		18		25	10	37	
0–19	23	24	74	62	31	18	9	5	0	10	2
Africa	5		100	39	18	23		0	13		
India	9	82	100	90	44	68	76	33	10	50	10
Japan	3	27	64	98	26	34	72	15	13	23	27

From Schroeder and Tipton (1968)

from Great Britain and America, the rise being particularly steep in the aorta, but this is not as evident in material from other countries (Figs 33–37).

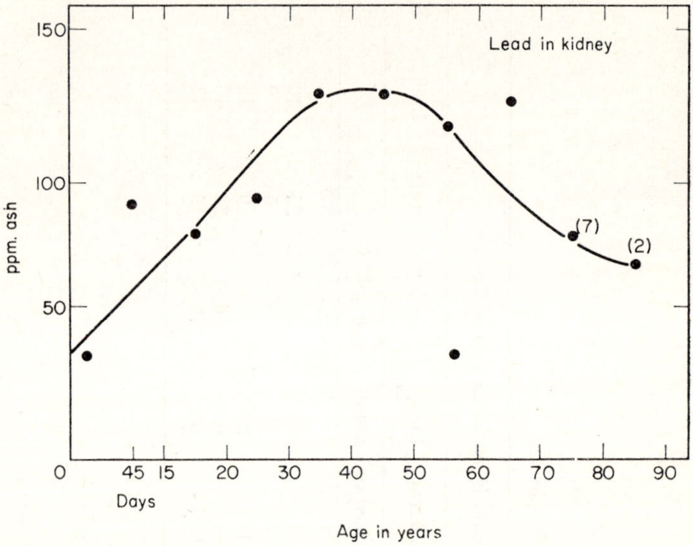

FIG. 33. Change in concentration of lead with age in kidney. Numbers in brackets in this and Figs 34–38 indicate number of cases in that decade when <9. Reproduced with permission from Schroeder and Balassa (1961).

C. Bone Lead

The skeleton contains by far the greatest proportion of lead in the body but is again subject to geographical variation (Table 30). Schroeder and Balassa (1961) have advanced some evidence that the concentration of lead in the bones rises consistently to the fourth decade when it remains relatively constant and then falls in the seventh and eighth decades (Table 31) (Fig. 38). Nusbaum *et al.* (1965) have also noted that bone lead concentrations were lowest at both extremes of age. This finding might be expected *a priori*, since the bones of the elderly often lose their mineral content and become osteoporotic and Hardy (1966) has even suggested that the mobilization of lead from the skeleton of elderly persons may be a cause of serious concern.

More recently, however, Barry (Barry and Mossman, 1970; Barry, 1972) has indicated that there is no fall in bone lead in extreme old age

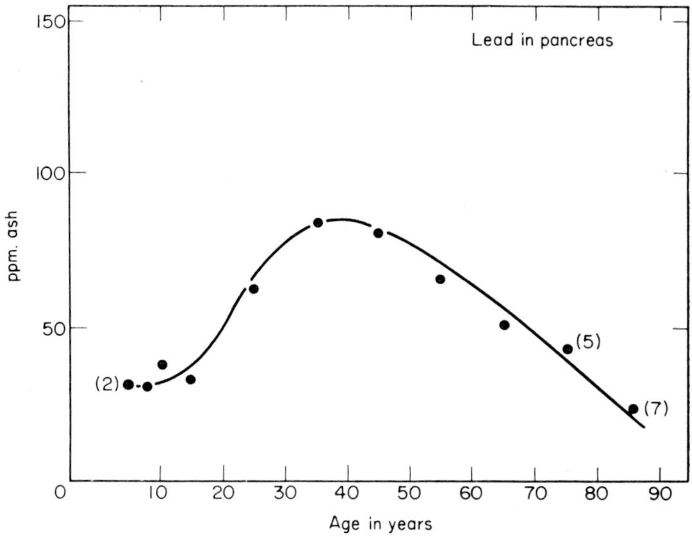

FIG. 34. Change in concentration of lead with age in pancreas. Reproduced with permission from Schroeder and Balassa (1961).

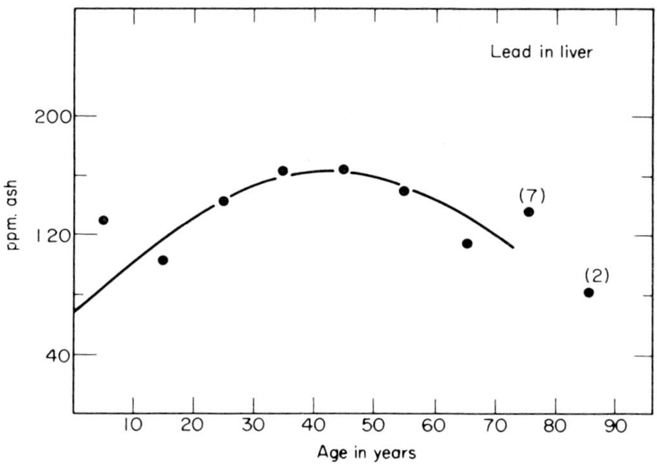

FIG. 35. Change in concentration of lead with age in liver. Reproduced with permission from Schroeder and Balassa (1961).

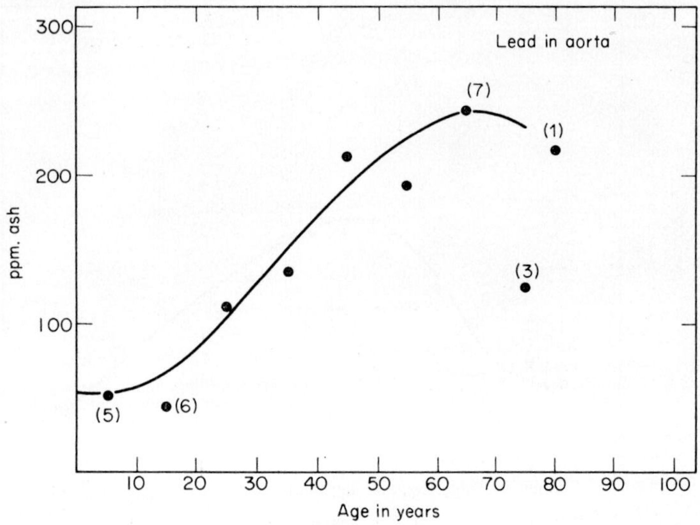

FIG. 36. Change in concentration of lead with age in aorta. Reproduced with permission from Schroeder and Balassa (1961).

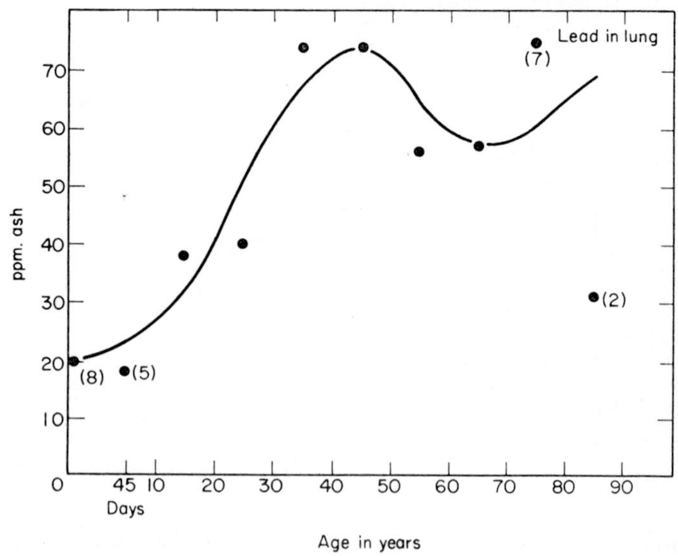

FIG. 37. Change in concentration of lead with age in lung. Reproduced with permission from Schroeder and Balassa (1961).

Table 31

Variation in bone lead concentration with age

Age (years)	n	Mean lead concentration µg/g ash
0–1	4	<1·0
1–9	2	2·5
10–19	9	11·3
20–29	11	16·8
30–39	27	43·1
40–49	9	37·2
50–59	9	31·2
60–69	5	34·2
70–79	2	10·0
80+	1	22·0

From Schroeder and Tipton (1968)

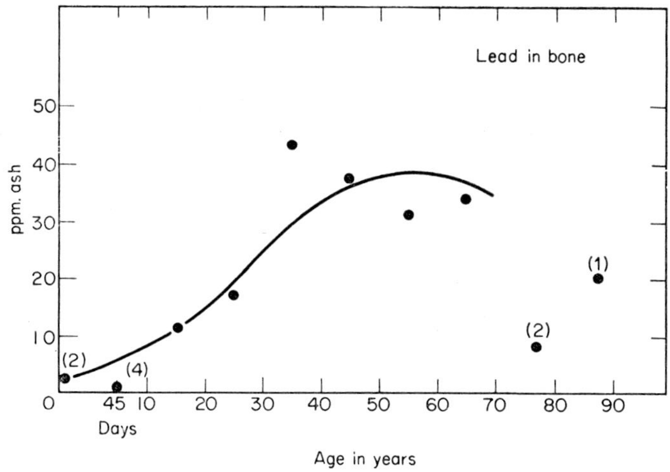

Fig. 38. Change in concentration of lead with age in bone. Reproduced with permission from Schroeder and Balassa (1961).

and suggested that the decline shown by the earlier workers was due to the small number of their samples. This is, in fact, confirmation of much earlier work by Morris (1940) who calculated regression coefficients between lead concentration in femur, rib and vertebrae and age. He found that lead content rose significantly with age and gave correlation coefficients of $r = 0{\cdot}48$, $0{\cdot}36$ and $0{\cdot}28$ respectively. He concluded from other data that more lead was stored in the long bones than either rib or the vertebrae, and most other authors have found lead to be distributed unevenly throughout the skeleton although they have not always agreed where the greatest concentration was to be found (Table 32). Holtzman

Table 32

Lead concentration in bone
micrograms Pb/g ash unless stated otherwise

Author	Flat bone	Rib	Long bone	Vertebra	Skull	Petrous
Kehoe *et al.* (1933b)	50–55		55			
Tompsett (1956)			76–540			
Henderson and Inglis (1957)		39 (M)			76 (M)	
		33 (F)			65 (F)	
Hill and Jaworowski (1961)			4·5[a]	6·6[a]		
Kehoe (1961a)	32		89			
Nusbaum *et al.* (1965)		69			69	
Becker *et al.* (1968)			50			
Jaworowski (1968)				3·9		
Schroeder and Tipton (1968)		47				
Barry and Mossmann (1970)		9[a] (M)	21[a] (M)			
		6[a] (F)	16[a] (F)			
Barry (1972)			26		24	41

[a] Micrograms Pb/g wet weight
M = males
F = females

(1963) has made a particularly exacting study of the concentration of lead (as naturally occurring ^{210}Pb) in the skeleton and has confirmed the variation from one bone to another. He demonstrated that the concentration of ^{210}Pb was higher in trabecular than in cortical bone and that the distribution could vary between different bones by as much as a factor of two. The skull bones seemed to be the most representative of the total skeleton since their concentration deviated least from the mean. Rib, by contrast, deviated most from the mean and was thought to represent the upper limit of skeletal lead concentration. The rather low figures in the tibia were considered to be due to the greater proportion of cortical bone present.

D. Hair Lead

Hair concentrates more lead per unit weight than any other tissue in the body (Bagchi *et al.*, 1940; Kraut and Weber, 1944; Goldblum *et al.*, 1953; Weinig and Börner, 1961). In common with a number of other heavy metals, lead is incorporated into hair protein in the follicle and is bound due to the presence of the abundant —SH groups in the follicular protein so that it is almost impossible to remove it (Bagchi *et al.*, 1940; Nishiyama, 1957). The amount of lead in the hair increases the further away the sample is from the scalp, indicating that lead is incorporated on the external surface from the atmosphere (Renshaw *et al.*, 1972).

Lead is normally present in the hair of healthy individuals but the concentration varies widely according to the diet and environment of the subject. Typical values have been quoted in the range from 2–284 μg/g (Flesch, 1954) but in the light of more recent work this second figure seems excessively high (Kopito *et al.*, 1967; Weiss *et al.*, 1972). It is for example, higher than the mean of the values found in workers in a lead battery plant (Nishiyama, 1957). Females have been reported as having higher hair lead concentrations than males (Tonomura *et al.*, 1965).

E. Total Body Burden

From an analysis of the tissues of one hundred and fifty Americans dying accidentally, Schroeder and Tipton (1968) calculated the total amount of lead in each organ. The total body burden found is shown in Table 33. The total body burden rises continually with age (Barry and Mossman, 1970) (Table 34).

Table 33

Variation in total body burden of lead with geographical location

Location	n	Total body burden (mg)
Nine American cities	150	121·6
San Francisco	27	137·2
Switzerland	9	61·9
Africa	54	63·2
Middle East	37	78·4
Far East	74	93·7

From Schroeder and Tipton (1968)

Table 34

Total body burden of lead by age and sex
Mean total body burden, mgPb

Age group	Male	*n*	Female	*n*
0–9	1·42	6	1·71	4
10–19	56·54	4		
20–29	85·51	5	30·59	3
30–39	178·60	3		
40–49	166·74	5	99·46	3
50–59	184·66	6	111·43	2
60–69	260·35	3	122·44	5
70–79			118·49	4
80+	265·71	3	172·80	3

From Barry and Mossman (1970)

3 Pathological Effects of Lead

I. EFFECTS ON HAEM SYNTHESIS

A. Normal Haem Synthesis

It is convenient to summarize the steps in haem synthesis. More detailed accounts may be found in the reviews of Tschudy (1969) and Dean (1971). The synthetic pathway is shown in Fig. 39.

Synthesis begins with the condensation of succinyl coenzyme A with glycine which has been activated by reaction with pyridoxal phosphate. The product of condensation, amino-keto-adipic acid is unstable and rapidly decarboxylates to form δ-aminolaevulinic acid (ALA). This initial reaction is catalysed by ALA synthetase (ALA-s). Two molecules of ALA condense to form porphobilinogen (PBG), the monopyrrollic precursor of the porphyrins. This step is catalysed by ALA dehydrase (ALA-d). From PBG, a polypyrrole of undetermined structure is formed by the action of PBG deaminase. This polypyrrole is probably not in the form of a closed ring, and a second enzyme, uroporphyrinogen III cosynthetase, is required to form uroporphyrinogen III which has eight carboxyl (COOH) groups in its molecule. When PBG deaminase acts on PBG in the absence of uroporphyrinogen III cosynthetase, uropophyrinogen I is formed. Uroporphyrinogen III is decarboxylated through a series of intermediates having six or five COOH groups to give coproporphyrinogen III, the reaction being catalysed by uroporphyrinogen decarboxylase. This enzyme can also act on uroporphyrinogen I to give coproporphyrinogen I.

Coproporphyrinogen III is converted to protoporphyrinogen by decarboxylation and oxidation reactions through the agency of two enzymes. The first, corproporphyrinogen oxidative decarboxylase catalyses the formation of protoporphyrinogen III whilst the second, protoporphyrinogen oxidase, converts protoporphyrinogen III to protoporphyrin III. The final step involves the chelation of ferrous iron to

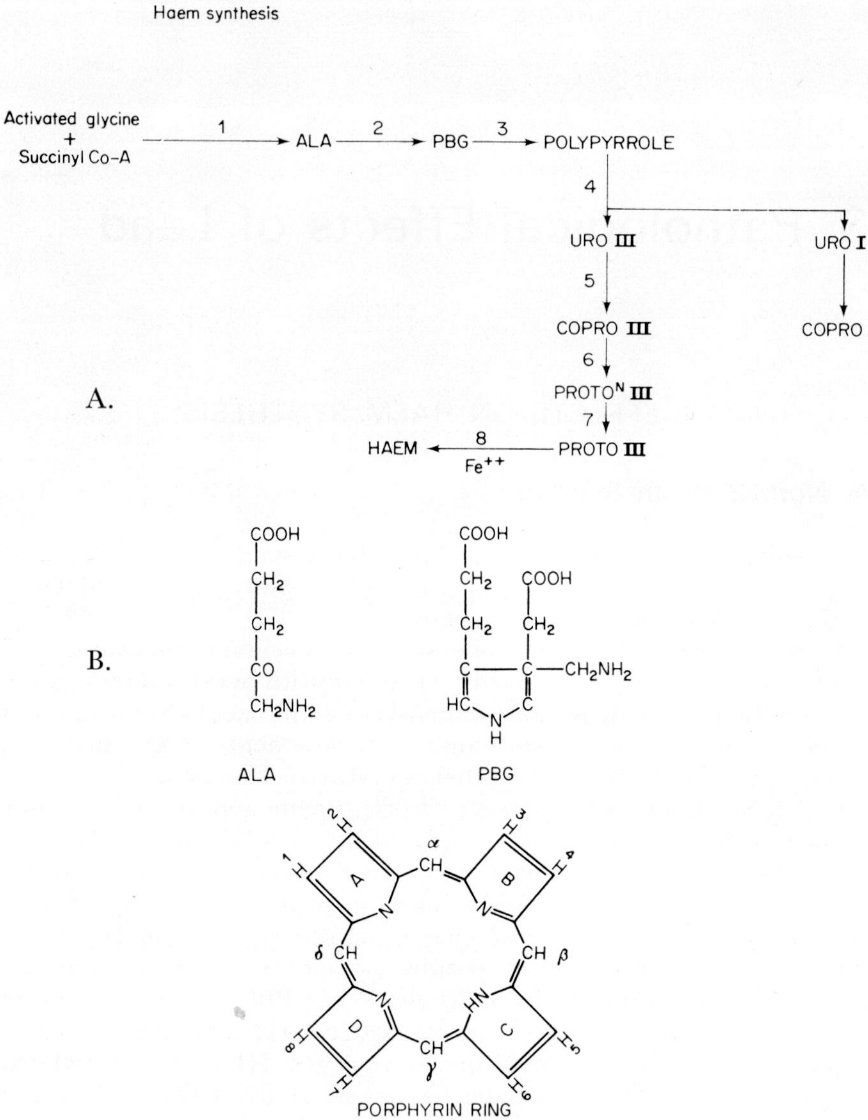

URO I	1, 3, 5, 7	CH_2COOH	2, 4, 6, 8	CH_2CH_2COOH
URO III	1, 3, 5, 8	CH_2COOH	2, 4, 6, 7	CH_2CH_2COOH
COPRO I	1, 3, 5, 7	CH_3	2, 4, 6, 8	CH_2CH_2COOH
COPRO III	1, 3, 5, 8	CH_3	2, 4, 6, 7	CH_2CH_2COOH
PROTO	1, 3, 5, 8	CH_3	2 4 $CH{=}CH_2$	6, 7 CH_2CH_2COOH

FIG. 39. A. Pathway of haem synthesis. *Abbreviations;* ALA δ-amino laevulinic acid; PBG porphobilinogen; URO uroporphyrinogen; COPRO coproporphyrinogen; PROTO[N] protoporphyrinogen; PROTO protoporphyrin. *Enzymes;* 1. ALA synthetase; 2. ALA dehydrase; 3. PBG deaminase (uroporphyrinogen I synthetase); 4. uroporphyrinogen III cosynthetase; 5. uroporphyrinogen decarboxylase; 6. coproporphyrinogen oxidative decarboxylase; 7. protoporphyrinogen oxidase; 8. haem synthetase (ferrochelatase). B. Formulae of haem precursors.

protoporphyrin to form haem. The enzyme responsible for this reaction is haem synthetase (ferrochelatase).

The enzymes involved in haem synthesis are compartmentalized within the cell. Those which mediate oxidation reactions, or which utilize oxidatively generated substrates are intramitochondrial. Those responsible for self-condensation reactions or decarboxylation are extramitochondrial (Fig. 40).

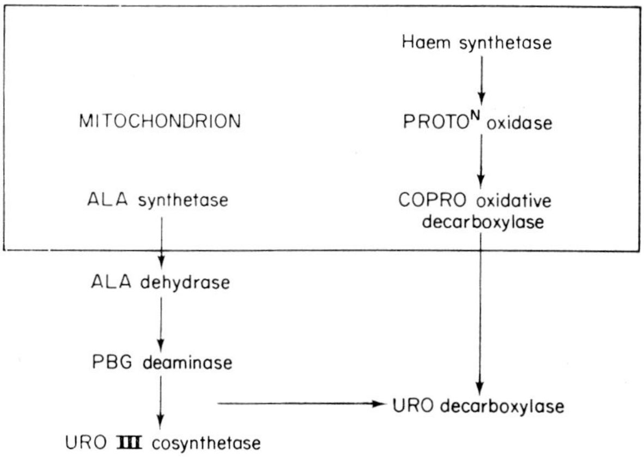

FIG. 40. Relation of enzymes involved in haem synthesis to the mitochondrion.

B. Effects of Lead

Since Garrod first demonstrated porphyrin in the urine in a case of lead poisoning in 1892 a great deal of attention has been given to the disturbances of haem synthesis which are caused by lead. The effects are summarized in Table 35.

Table 35

Changes in the concentration of porphyrins and their precursors in lead poisoning

	Blood RBC's	Blood Plasma	Urine	Faeces
ALA		+	+++	
PBG		N	±−+	
URO	±	N	±−+	N
COPRO	+	±	+++	N
PROTO	+++	±	N−±	N

N = normal

1. *ALA and PBG*

The urinary excretion of ALA is markedly raised in lead poisoning and its appearance in increased amounts is an early sign of metabolic lead poisoning in adults (Tishkoff *et al.*, 1958; Haeger-Aronsen, 1960; Holmqvist, 1960; de Kretser and Waldron, 1963a; Gattner and Schrantz, 1964). There is disagreement as to whether ALA excretion is an early and dependable sign of poisoning in children, some authorities stating that it is (Davis *et al.*, 1968; Vitale *et al.*, 1972) others (Blumenthal *et al.*, 1972) holding the contrary view.

Raised urinary ALA concentrations are closely correlated with plasma levels which are elevated prior to the urinary increase (Haeger-Aronson, 1960; Danieli *et al.*, 1961; Rasetti and Parigi, 1962; Chiesura and Brugnone, 1963; Albahary, 1964, 1972; Saita and Moreo, 1967; Waldron, unpublished data). With low levels of lead exposure there is considerable variation in ALA excretion which becomes a function of urine osmolality (Barnes *et al.*, 1972).

The methods most often used to measure ALA concentration in fact measure total amino-ketones which in the urine are mainly ALA and amino-acetone. Amino-acetone excretion increases with increased ALA excretion in men exposed to lead (Waldron, 1965) and in persons with lead poisoning (Meo *et al.*, 1964; Pisani *et al.*, 1967) although some workers have reported findings to the contrary (Schlenker *et al.*, 1964, Druyan and Haeger-Aronsen, 1964). The position regarding PBG excretion is also unclear and there has been controversy as to whether urinary excretion is, or is not, raised in lead workers and in cases of frank plumbism. In lead workers it is only moderately if at all raised, and even in cases of severe plumbism the levels of excretion are inconsiderable (Watson *et al.*, 1953; Bashour, 1954, Tishkoff *et al.*, 1958; Griggs and Harris, 1958; Tanabe, 1959; Haeger-Aronsen, 1960; de Kretser and Waldron, 1963a; de Bruin and Holboom, 1967; Gibson *et al.*, 1968; Berk *et al.*, 1970; Gibson and Goldberg, 1970; de Bruin, 1971; Albahary, 1972). Plasma levels are invariably normal (Waldron, unpublished data).

2. *Porphyrins*

a. Urine. Coproporphyrin, mainly isomer III, is excreted in excess in the urine of persons exposed to lead and in cases of plumbism, although not invariably in children (Moncrieff *et al.*, 1964; Griggs, 1964; Moosa and Harris, 1969; Betts *et al.*, 1973). It was the earliest biochemical abnormality discovered in lead poisoning and its use as a screening method for workers in lead industries has long been advocated (de Langen and ten Berg, 1948; Maloof, 1950; Brooks, 1951; Pinto *et al.*, 1952; Wyllie, 1955).

Other porphyrins are not present in the urine to such a great extent although protoporphyrin may occasionally be detected in increased amount (Waldron, unpublished data) and so may uroporphyrin (Bashour, 1954), especially in severe cases of lead poisoning (Stanković *et al.*, 1972). In a few cases porphyrins containing three or six COOH groups have been found by chromatographic methods (Waldron, 1964a).

b. Blood. The most notable finding is a greatly increased concentration of erythrocyte protoporphyrin (Vigliani and Angeleri, 1935; Watson, 1950; Rubino *et al.*, 1958; Byers, 1959; Rubino, 1962; Sano *et al.*, 1960; Beattie *et al.*, 1972a; Albahary, 1972) especially during the acute stages of intoxication (Byers, 1959) although elevated levels have been found up to three years after exposure to lead has ceased (Rubino *et al.*, 1958). It is a particularly useful sign in children (Watson *et al.*, 1958; Nelson *et al.*, 1968) and a recent simple method using capillary blood as a screening procedure has been recommended by Kammholz *et al.* (1972). An equally effective screening test has been suggested by Whitaker and Vietti (1958), who have shown that the increased protoporphyrin causes from 75–100 per cent of the red cells from cases of childhood plumbism to fluoresce under the ultra-violet microscope.

The coproporphyrin content of the red cells may also be greater than normal (Schmid *et al.*, 1950; Rubino *et al.*, 1960; Waldron, unpublished data) although it may decrease in the later stages of the disease (Chisolm, 1964). Plasma porphyrins may be slightly elevated mainly due to an increase in protoporphyrin content (Waldron, 1964a), but raised coproporphyrin levels have also been described (Sano, 1958).

c. Faeces. Faecal porphyrins are invariably normal in lead poisoning (Haeger-Aronsen, 1962).

3. *Effects on Enzymes Concerned with Haem Synthesis*

a. Haem synthetase. It was Rimington (1937) who first suggested that lead might prevent the incorporation of iron into the propoporphyrin molecule and this theory has been adequately substantiated. At a concentration of about 10^{-4} M lead produces a profound inhibition in the enzyme *in vitro* (Rimington, 1956; Dresel and Falk, 1956; Goldberg *et al.*, 1956; Gibson and Goldberg, 1970) and the effect diminishes thereafter with diminishing concentration (Gajdos-Török *et al.*, 1960; Klein, 1962). The inhibiting effect has also been found *in vivo* in patients suffering from lead poisoning (Boyett and Butterworth, 1962). According to Otrzonsek (1967) the inhibiting effect is most noted in the bone marrow but conversely liver cells show an increased activity which enables them to take over some part of haem synthesis.

b. ALA-d. ALA-d activity was shown experimentally to be inhibited by lead and other metals with an affinity for —SH groups (Gibson *et al.*, 1955; Granick and Mauzerall, 1958). Further studies have shown that the activity of the enzyme is inhibited *in vivo* in experimental animals, in lead workers and in cases of plumbism (Rubino, 1962; Lichtman and Feldman, 1963; Bonsignore *et al.*, 1965; Bonsignore, 1966; de Bruin, 1968; Nakao *et al.*, 1968; Hernberg *et al.*, 1970, 1972; Millar *et al.*, 1970; Giménez *et al.*, 1970; Hernberg and Nikkanen, 1970; Haeger-Aronsen *et al.*, 1971). In lead poisoning ALA-d activity is inhibited in brain, liver, kidney, bone marrow, and erythrocytes. The addition of glutathione restores activity to kidney and bone marrow homogenates but there is still marked inhibition in brain and liver (Gibson and Goldberg, 1970).

ALA-d is very sensitive to the effects of lead, and inhibition of the enzyme is observed in city dwellers with no industrial exposure and the inhibitory effect correlates well with the blood lead concentration (Hernberg and Nikkanen, 1970). The measurement of the enzyme activity in circulating red cells is a sensitive index of lead poisoning and has been used to screen children for the disease (Weissberg *et al.*, 1971).

c. ALA-synthetase. Although it had been reported that the activity of this enzyme was unaffected by lead (Pecora *et al.*, 1964; Gajdos and Gajdos-Török, 1964) it is now established that progressive inhibition is found with increasing lead concentration. The effect is more marked in anaerobic conditions (Rubino, 1961; Morrow *et al.*, 1969).

d. Effects on other enzymes. Using radio-isotope techniques in the rabbit, Kreiner-Birnbaum and Grinstein (1965) were able to show that uroporphyrinogen decarboxylase and coproporphyrinogen decarboxylase are both inhibited to some degree by lead.

e. Other effects. Ericksen (1955) has suggested that globin synthesis may be adversely affected whilst Albahary (1972) has put forward the view that the incorporation of iron into protoporphyrin, for which glutathione is required, might be secondarily affected as a consequence of the low glutathione concentrations found in the blood in lead poisoning. This author also considered that the transaminase which is involved in the synthesis of purine from ALA might be inhibited, thus making more ALA available for porphyrin synthesis (Albahary, 1972).

f. Summary. There may be at least five stages in haem synthesis which lead inhibits (Fig. 41). The enzymes catalysing stages one, four and five are situated within the mitochondrion.

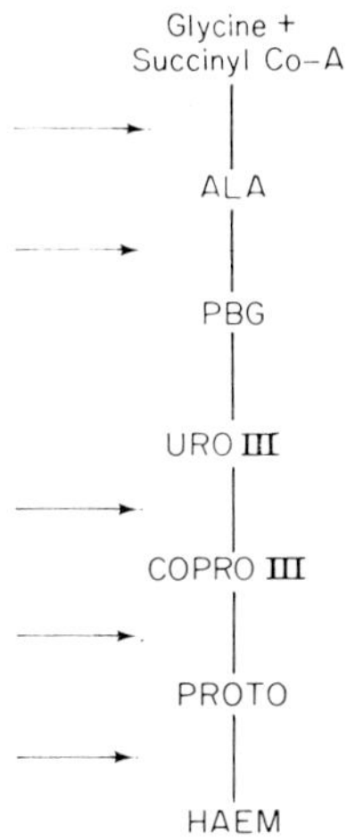

FIG. 41. Stages of haem synthesis inhibited by lead (arrows).

4. *Porphyrin Synthesis in TEL Poisoning*

Porphyrin metabolism is not deranged in organic lead poisoning to the same extent as in inorganic poisoning. ALA and PBG levels in the urine are normal but coproporphyrin excretion may be slightly raised (Beattie *et al.*, 1972c). Erythrocyte protoporphyrin concentrations are not raised except in severe cases (Gutniak *et al.*, 1964; Beattie *et al.*, 1972c).

ALA-d activity, however, is significantly decreased in the red cells of men working with lead alkyls and in cases of clinical poisoning (Millar *et al.*, 1972; Beattie *et al.*, 1972c). Millar's group found that diethyl lead was also able to inhibit the enzyme but to a lesser degree than Pb^{++} ions.

5. *Comparison with the Porphyrias*

The symptoms of inorganic lead poisoning have many similarities with those of acute intermittent porphyria (AIP) (Dagg *et al.*, 1965), but biochemically the conditions are distinct. The basic defect in AIP is the increase of ALA-s activity in the liver and this is the first overproduction disease described where the defect can be localized to a single enzyme (Tschudy *et al.*, 1965). There is no such induction of ALA-s in the liver in lead poisoned animals (Gajdos and Gajdos-Török, 1971). Again by contrast with lead poisoning, the main metabolite in the urine in the hepatic prophyrias is PBG which may be present even in remissions.

The erythropoietic porphyrias are characterized by increased erythrocyte protoporphyrin, but the main urinary porphyrin is uroporphyrin although coproporphyrin is also present, but ALA and PBG are not excreted in excess. There are no abdominal or neurological symptoms referable to erythropoietic porphyria and conversely, sensitization to sunlight does not occur in lead poisoning.

There seems little justification, therefore, to regard the common symptomatology of AIP and lead poisoning as anything more than coincidental and it is not indicative of a common underlying metabolic disorder.

II. IRON METABOLISM

There have been a large number of reports of raised serum iron concentrations with a lowered total iron binding capacity (TIBC) in lead poisoning (Vanotti and Imholz, 1939; Prader, 1948; Grazianni *et al.*, 1954, 1956; Larizza and Ventura, 1954; Saita *et al.*, 1955; Rubino *et al.*, 1958; Tishkoff *et al.*, 1958; Hutchinson and Stark, 1961; David, 1963; Zegarski, 1963) and in addition, plasma iron kinetics are altered. Iron is cleared from the plasma at an increased rate together with the total iron flux through the plasma (Beck *et al.*, 1955; Boyett and Butterworth, 1962; Paolino *et al.*, 1963; Simpson *et al.*, 1964; Sroczyński *et al.*, 1964, 1966; Berk *et al.*, 1970). There have been reports that this is not always so in children. Leikin and Eng (1963) studied seven children with plumbism and found that plasma iron clearance time was prolonged in the three with the longest history of exposure and that the rate of incorporation of iron into the red cells was decreased. The four children with the shortest exposure were found to have normal or increased iron-turnover results.

The rate of iron utilization by the red cells has been reported as being both decreased (Boyett *et al.*, 1960; Boyett and Butterworth, 1962; Simpson *et al.*, 1964) and increased (Sroczyński *et al.*, 1964; Berk *et al.*, 1970).

Jandl *et al.* (1959) showed that the uptake of ^{59}Fe by human reticulocytes was almost completely inhibited by the addition of 5×10^{-4}M Pb^{2+} but that the inhibition was less marked at lower concentrations. The incorporation of ^{59}Fe into haemoglobin was also almost entirely prevented with the consequence that the amount of iron in the red-cell membrane was greatly increased. Reticulocytes from bled rabbits incubated with 10^{-4} M Pb^{2+} showed only a moderate dimunition of cellular uptake of ^{59}Fe but there was a striking increase in the amount of iron in the stromal fraction of hydrolysed centrifuged cells, confirming earlier reports of an accumulation of iron in the stroma of immature red cells in cases of human plumbism (Bessis and Breton-Gorius, 1957c). Later, Allen and Jandl (1960) extended their investigations using washed rabbit reticulocytes. They found that iron taken into these cells was associated with various particulate fractions, being released to become incorporated into a transient non-haemoglobin protein phase and finally forming part of the haemoglobin molecule. They found that lead allowed iron to accumulate in the particulate fractions but that it blocked its entry into the non-haemoglobin protein and also into haemoglobin. This was confirmed by Lothe and Falbe-Hansen (1963) who concluded that lead blocked the transfer of iron from a ferritin phase to a mitochondrial fraction.

The increased intracellular iron can be demonstrated by the electron microscope and may be associated with the mitochondria (Bessis and Breton-Gorius, 1957a, b, c, d, 1959; Bessis, 1958; Pernis and Bairati, 1959; Pernis *et al.*, 1959, 1964; Jensen *et al.*, 1965; Albahary, 1972) (Fig. 42). Bessis and Jensen (1965) say that two types of non-haem iron may be found inside the abnormal sideorblast from the bone marrow of lead-poisoned animals and from patients with plumbism, ferritin, similar to that found in normal cells, and an abnormal type of iron which they term ferruginous miscelles. These are either dust-like or they occur in plaques having no constant form. Ferritin is found within the mitochondria whereas it is only found in the cytoplasm of normal cells. An increase in intra-cellular iron is shown by the increased numbers of siderocytes found in the peripheral blood (Albahary, 1972).

The electron microscope also shows that the structure of the normoblast is severely altered, reflecting, perhaps, the high concentration of lead found in the bone marrow (Westerman *et al.*, 1965). The nuclear membrane may be thinned but most of the changes occur in the cytoplasmic organelles. The Golgi apparatus is swollen and the mitochondria appear grossly enlarged and their crisae are disorganized although they still show their typical double membrane (Jensen *et al.*, 1965).

Several stages of haem synthesis are known to be facilitated by intact mitochondriae (Sano, 1958; Sano *et al.*, 1959; Bessis and Jensen, 1965) and it has been suggested that they may function as an intermediary in intracellular iron metabolism (Cooper *et al.*, 1963). They are probably necessary for the continued transfer of iron from extracellular sites to normoblasts of reticulocytes (Jandl *et al.*, 1959; Morgan and Laurell,

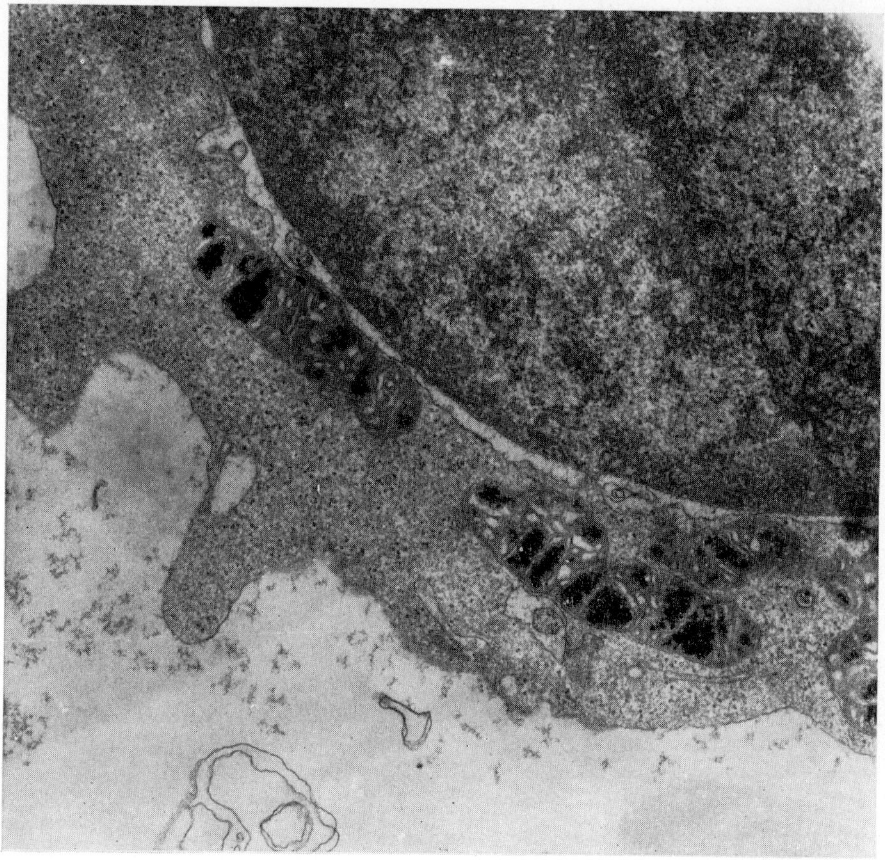

FIG. 42. EM of part of a polychromatic erythroblast from the bone marrow of a patient with lead poisoning. Mitochondria are seen containing ferruginous miscelles and showing distension of the intercristal spaces. The perinuclear canal is dilated and there is decreased polyribosome formation. × 22500.

1963) and the altered appearance of the mitochondria in these cells in lead poisoning indicates a further mechanism whereby lead interferes with haem synthesis.

The accumulation of iron within the normoblast may itself interfere with haem synthesis. Morrow *et al.* (1969) have shown that high concentrations of ferrous iron (10^{-3} M) inhibit the action of ALA synthetase and they have suggested that this may be the mechanism whereby certain refractory anaemias are aggravated by the administration of excess iron (Verloop *et al.*, 1962; Harris *et al.*, 1965). Thus lead could have two effects of this enzyme, first a direct inhibition and second, an indirect inhibition resulting from the accumulation of iron within the mitochondria.

Berk *et al.* (1970) showed in their single case that iron kinetics return to normal after treatment (Table 36).

Table 36

Changes in iron kinetics after treatment in a case of lead poisoning

	Before treatment	After treatment
$T\frac{1}{2}$ plasma ^{59}Fe (min)	45	95
Total iron flux through plasma (mg/24 hr)	73·4	25·2
Plasma iron turnover (mg/24 hr)	36·6	19·8
Red cell ^{59}Fe utilization (% of dose)	73·8	80·0
Red cell iron turnover (mg/24 hr)	27·0	80·0

From Berk *et al.* (1970)

III. THE ANAEMIA

The anaemia of lead poisoning is seldom severe although a profound fall in haemoglobin has been reported and was common when there was a vogue for treating malignant disease with intravenous lead injections (Bell *et al.*, 1925; Brookfield, 1928; Withers, 1930; Gould *et al.*, 1937). It is usually a hypochromic and normocytic anaemia although macrocytosis may develop if the anaemia persists for any length of time (Saita *et al.*, 1952). In children, the anaemia is usually more severe and more pronouncedly microcytic and hypochromic perhaps because lead poisoning in children is often coincidentally associated with a nutritional iron-deficiency state (Watson *et al.*, 1958).

The anaemia of lead poisoning has many characteristics in common with thalassaemia and it must be differentiated from this condition. Patients known to have thalassaemia should not be exposed to lead (Albahary, 1972). The differentiation of thalassaemia from lead poisoning lies in demonstrating the presence of haemoglobin A_2 which in patients with thalassaemia may be present in amounts up to 10 per cent, whereas normally it represents less than 3 per cent of total haemoglobin. Foetal haemoglobin (HbF) may constitute 40–90 per cent of the total in thalassaemia but it has also been reported in excess in lead poisoning although in only a very few cases (Buczkowski, 1964; Albahary, 1972). Haemoglobin A_2 is also occasionally increased, and in babies with severe poisoning "HbPb", a haemoglobin similar to HbA_3, has been reported (Tuttle and Fitch, 1958, Charache and Weatherall, 1966). This subject is well reviewed by Albahary (1972).

The attention of most of the early workers was drawn to the basophilic stippled cell and its production (Legge and Goadby, 1912; Oliver, 1914; Price-Jones, 1924–25). The connection between these cells and cells containing iron-staining inclusion bodies was also much discussed (MacFadzean and Davies, 1947, 1949). Dustin (1943, 1944) showed that the basophilic material in the stippled cells was a ribonuclear protein and Jensen and his colleagues (Jensen and Moreno, 1964; Jensen *et al.*; 1965) showed by extensive electron micrograph studies, that these cells were reticulocytes and that the differing appearances between stippled cells and reticulocytes were largely due to the different manipulations involved in preparing films for examination under the optical microscope. Beritić (1963) showed that stippled cells and siderocytes were separate entities although iron-staining inclusion bodies could co-exist in cells together with basophilic staining material. Basophilic stippling occurs in such a wide variety of conditions beside lead poisoning, for example in many haemolytic anaemias, thalassaemia, leukaemia, and after exposure to aniline, arsenic, benzene, carbon monoxide and copper, that it is nowadays regarded as an unreliable index of lead absorption (Griggs, 1964), and the discussions which so occupied workers thirty to forty years ago are now of little but historical interest.

The production of lead anaemia is complex. There is no doubt that alterations in haem synthesis and iron metabolism play a considerable part, but the role of a haemolytic mechanism is still open to debate (Waldron, 1966).

Aub and Reznikoff (1924) proposed a scheme whereby lead rendered the red cell more liable to mechanical trauma during passage through the capillaries. According to them lead combined with the inorganic phosphate on the red cell membrane with the local release of hydrochloric acid

$$3PbCl_2 + 2Na_2HPO_4 = Pb_3(PO_4)_2 + 4NaCl + 2HCl.$$

They found that leaded red cells shaken in a tonometer were less resistant to mechanical trauma than normal cells, and this observation has been reported also by some other workers (Sutherland and Eisentraut, 1956; Fratianne *et al.*, 1959; Harris and Greenberg, 1954). On the other hand, a number of workers have shown the mechanical fragility to be normal in lead poisoning (Baron, 1954; Rubino *et al.*, 1956; de Kretser and Waldron, 1963b; Griggs, 1964). De Kretser and Waldron (1965) found that there was no increase in the mechanical fragility of cells leaded *in vitro* until the concentration of lead was greater than 10 μg/ml and that at a concentration of 45 μgPb^{2+}/ml saturation was reached and the addition of more lead did not result in a further increase in fragility.

There is a considerable increase in mechanical fragility if leaded red cells are incubated for 24 hr (Waldron, 1964b) but it seems unlikely that an increase in mechanical fragility contributes significantly to the production of lead anaemia. Nor is there any confirmation that free acid is produced on the red cell membrane, and, indeed, there is evidence that it is not so formed (Maxwell and Bischoff, 1929a, b).

Studies on the life-span of the erythrocyte using Ashby's differential agglutination technique (Ashby, 1921) or tagging with ^{51}Cr have yielded equivocal results and both normal and abnormal results have been reported (Sheets *et al.*, 1951; Crepet *et al.*, 1956; Griggs and Harris, 1958; Rubino *et al.*, 1959; Fratianne *et al.*, 1959; Goldberg, 1960; Hutchinson and Stark, 1961; Leikin and Eng, 1963; Combrisson *et al.*, 1964; Simpson *et al.*, 1964). There are serious theoretical disadvantages to using ^{51}Cr as a marker, however, in particular the continuous and variable elution of the isotope from circulating labelled cells results in a continuously changing rate of disappearance of the label (Eadie *et al.*, 1960; Cline and Berlin, 1963a). Moreover, the toxic effect of chromate and the effect of ionizing radiation from the isotope increase the difficulties (Hernberg, 1967). Using tritiated di-isopropylfluorophosphonate (^{3}H-DFP) seems to overcome most of these limitations (Cline and Berlin, 1963a, b). Hernberg and his colleagues (Hernberg, 1967; Hernberg *et al.*, 1967a) have used this label to demonstrate a decrease in red cell life span in cases of frank poisoning and in men with considerable industrial exposure but no symptoms.

In considering a decrease in red cell life span, two mechanisms may be distinguished (Berlin *et al.*, 1959). The cells may be destroyed either by premature senescence, resulting in a true shortening of life span, in which case the effect is non-random and all cells of equal age disappear from the circulation at the same time. The rate of disappearance of a label from the population is

$$N_t = N_0\left(1 - \frac{t}{T}\right)$$

where N_0 and N_t equal the specific activity of the cells (or the number of circulating labelled cells) at zero time and time t. T equals the life span of the cells. The rate of disappearance of label will be a linear function. Alternatively, there may be increased random destruction of the cells which is independent of cell age. In this case the life span is potentially normal but some process acts upon the cell causing it to disappear prematurely, and the rate of disappearance is an exponential function following the expression

$$N_t = N_0 e^{-kt}$$

where *k* equals the fraction of radioactivity removed in unit time. In Hernberg's studies the destruction was non-random, indicating that lead was acting to shorten the true life span of the red cell, although the mechanism of this action was not clear. By contrast, Berk *et al.* (1970), in the exhaustive study they made of a single case, found random shortening of the life-span.

Thus, it does seem proven that lead causes a shortening of red cell life be it random or non-random. The means by which it achieves this is not yet certain although it is likely to be due to a direct effect on the integrity of the red cell membrane. There is a leakage of potassium from erythrocytes when they are incubated with lead, an effect which is also noted in cells taken from men exposed to lead industrially (Joyce *et al.*, 1954; Grigarzik and Passow, 1958; Passow *et al.*, 1961; Hernberg, 1967; Hasan *et al.*, 1967a). In addition, red cell adenosine triphosphatase (ATP-ase) is reduced together with an increase in cell ATP (Hasan and Hernberg, 1966; Hasan *et al.*, 1967b; Hernberg *et al.*, 1967a, b, c; Secchi *et al.*, 1968; Gajdos and Gajdos-Török, 1971). The effect on the membrane is an early response to lead and appears long before clinical symptoms are obvious. There is also an effect on the uptake of ^{32}P by the cells, which is reduced in men having severe exposure to lead (Rozenberg and Smirnova, 1961; Westerman and Jensen, 1963). The membrane ATP-ase levels return to normal when exposure to lead is discontinued or treatment with EDTA has been instigated (Secchi *et al.*, 1968).

It is reasonable to suppose that membrane effects are sufficient to alter the life span of the red cell, although there is in addition, evidence that the internal metabolism of the cell is adversely affected. The rate of glucose utilization by red cells is slightly increased in persons with lead exposure and is correlated to coproporphyrin excretion (Hasan and Hernberg, 1966; Hernberg *et al.*, 1967b).

Although haemolytic mechanism does contribute towards the production of lead anaemia the changes in red cell life span are not great and it is incorrect to label the anaemia as predominantly haemolytic in type. Haptoglobin levels are normal (Sroczyński and Kossman, 1966) but the Coombs test has been reported as positive in experimental animals and in cases of human plumbism (Sutherland and Eisentraut, 1956; Crutcher, 1963). Other authors report a negative result (Fullerton, 1952; Tishkoff *et al.*, 1958; Karpatkin, 1961; Rickword-Lane and Lawrence, 1961; Simpson *et al.*, 1964; Fromke *et al.*, 1969; Desoille *et al.*, 1970). If the red cells from lead workers are separated and the fraction rich in reticulocytes is tested, then a positive reaction is found (Sutherland and Eisentraut, 1956; Pernis and Finulli, 1960) suggesting that either the transferrin present on the surface of the immature cells produces the effect, or lead, in combination with a protein on the cell surface of the reticulocytes (stippled cells) forms a hapten which can lead to agglutination in the presence of Coombs' serum (Jandl, 1960).

IV. THE NERVOUS SYSTEM

Neurological symptoms attributable to lead poisoning have been recognized since antiquity. Both the peripheral and the central nervous systems may be affected and changes in the anterior horn cells of the spinal cord have also been reported resulting in a syndrome not unlike motor neurone disease.

A. Peripheral Nerves

The earliest extensive study of the histological abnormalities found in lead neuropathy was made by Gombault (1880). He observed both degenerative and regenerative changes in the myelin sheaths of guinea pigs which had developed a peripheral neuropathy as the result of chronic lead intoxication. Gombault found that the myelin sheaths disintegrated in a segmental fashion beginning at the node of Ranvier; but that after, or even during, the removal of the disintegrating sheaths, short segments of myelin were restored. In contrast to the extensive damage done to the myelin sheaths, Gombault found that the axon was unaffected.

Gombault's results with respect to the damage to the myelin sheaths have since been confirmed, but it seems likely that he was in error in stating that the axon remains intact in lead neuropathy. In a study of 52 guinea pigs with chronic lead intoxication, Fullerton (1966) found histological abnormalities in the peripheral nerves of 31, although in none was there any clinical signs of neurological abnormality. The most common change seen in the peripheral nerves of these animals was a mixture of segmental demyelination and axonal degeneration (18/31). In a further 8 animals segmental demyelination alone was found and in another 5, axonal degeneration was present in the absence of any demyelination. These results are clearly in disagreement with those of Gombault but receive confirmation from later studies by Schlaepfer (1968) and Lampert and Schochet (1968) who used chronically lead-poisoned rats as their experimental model. In both the last two cases, however, axonal degeneration was far less frequently encountered than segmental demyelination (Fig. 43).

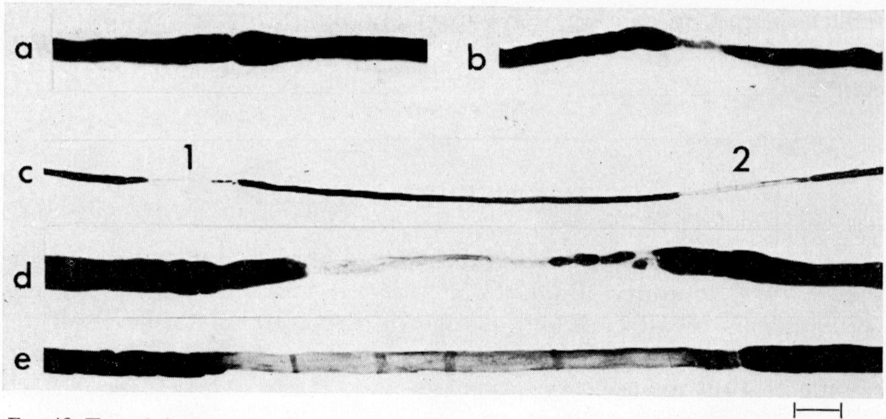

FIG. 43. Teased single nerves fibres stained with 1 per cent osmium tetroxide to show various stages of segmental demyelination. a. Normal node of Ranvier. b. Widened node from lead poisoned animal. c. Fibre from poisoned animal to show short length of demyelination (1) and remyelination of previously demyelinated region (2). d. Demyelinated region 1 at higher magnification. e. Remyelinated region 2 at higher magnification. Bar = 20 μ for a, b, d, e, 75 μ for c. Reproduced with permission from Fullerton (1964).

The earliest change which Fullerton noted in her experimental animals was a widening of the node of Ranvier. This change is not peculiar to lead neuropathy having also been noted as an early feature of diphtheritic neuropathy (Waksman *et al.*, 1957; Webster *et al.*, 1961; Cavanagh and Jacobs, 1964; Jacobs *et al.*, 1966), and in the neuropathies induced by x-irradiation (Andres, 1963; Massurovsky *et al.*, (1967) or spinal barbotage (Bunge *et al.*, 1960). The process of demyelination, which begins at the node of Ranvier, may stop before it involves the whole internode and a phase of remyelination may then supervene with no change in the length of the internode. On the other hand, if the whole internode *is* affected, then recovery results in the formation of several short segments and a number of new nodes. Different stages of demyelination and remyelination may be found in the same animal, often even in the same nerve fibre.

Fullerton found several nerve fibres to be undergoing axonal degeneration and large ovoids of degenerating myelin, indistinguishable from the Wallerian degeneration seen after axotomy, were seen in sections stained with osmic acid. In silver-stained preparations, the axons showed a fragmented appearance. There was a marked decrease in the number of fibres of large diameter but no decrease in the number of fibres of small diameter. It was suggested that this might be due to a relative increase in the number of small-diameter fibres due to the plane of section passing through regions where large-diameter fibres were undergoing remyelination after first having had their sheaths disrupted.

During the course of her investigations, Fullerton also examined a small number of rats with an induced lead neuropathy, noting in these animals, in contrast to the guinea pig, only scanty change in the nerve fibres, thus confirming earlier work by other authors (Prevost and Binet, 1927). In the studies of Schlaepfer (1968), and Lampert and Schochet (1968), however, severe demyelination was observed in rats with lead neuropathy, morphologically similar to that reported by Fullerton in the guinea pig. The disparity between these various sets of results is difficult to explain, but since both the later studies were more exhaustive than Fullerton's and supported by electron microscope findings (*vide infra*), the balance of evidence must be weighted in their favour.

It is important to note, however, that a considerable species variation exists regarding the proportion of segmental demyelination to axonal degeneration in animals with lead neuropathy (Hopkins, 1970). For example, axonal degeneration is found more commonly than demyelination in rabbits (Doinikow, 1911; Shimazono, 1914; de Villaverde, 1929–1930). In humans, also, axonal degeneration seems to be the predominant lesion (Herter, 1895), segmental demyelination having never been described, although specifically looked for by at least two groups of workers (Laslett and Warrington, 1898; Phillippe and Gothard, 1903). In cats, on the other hand, very scanty axonal degeneration or demyelination is found in peripheral nerves although these animals rapidly become paralysed after exposure to lead salts (Legge and Goadby, 1912), and in this species, the changes seem to be mainly confined to the central nervous system (Ferraro and Hernandez, 1932).

With the electron microscope, the earliest changes seen in the Schwann cell are at the nodes of Ranvier or the Schmidt-Lantermann clefts and these manifest themselves as a separation and an irregular infolding of the myelin lamellae resulting in a marked disturbance of the tubular configuration of the sheath. Membranes derived from detached myelin form small bodies partially filling the spaces between the separated lamellae. At the nodes of Ranvier the terminal cytoplasmic loops of the myelin lamellae are either swollen, or collapsed and transformed into granular buds (Schlaepfer, 1968; Lampert and Schochet, 1968) (Fig. 44).

Regeneration of the myelin sheath is manifested by the presence of Schwann cells which can be seen undergoing mitosis and by the presence of a large number of Schwann cell processes covering both normal and abnormal sheaths.

After the myelin debris has been removed from about the axon, proliferating Schwann cells grow around the denuded axon, and new myelin lamellae are formed by the fusion of the inner surfaces of the plasma membranes of the spirally wrapped Schwann cell processes. The

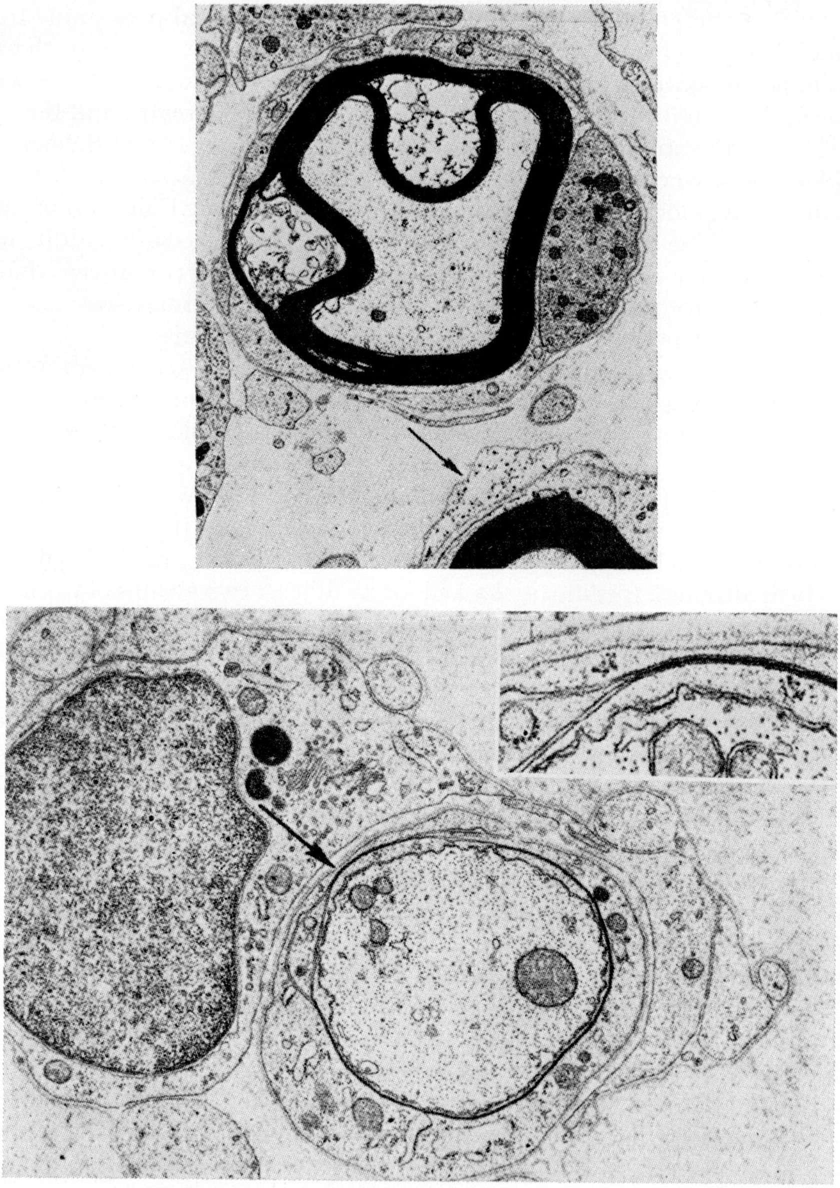

FIG. 44. A. Myelinated axons from lead poisoned rat. Upper myelin sheath shows wide disruptions and vesicular breakdown of lamellae. Both sheaths are surrounded by proliferated Schwann processes, some of which are degenerating (arrow), ×8,000. B. Remyelination in an axon, ×12,000. Inset (arrowed) shows a single myelin lamella formed by the fusion of Schwann cell plasma membranes, ×30,000. Reproduced with permission from Lampert and Schochet (1968).

basement lamina of the Schwann cell forms a new neurolemmal tube for the axon.

An additional finding noted only by Lampert and Schochet (1968) is the presence of "onion bulbs" around the axons caused by the repeated degeneration and regeneration of Schwann cells. This finding is of interest because it is reminiscent of the same phenomenon seen in some human neuropathies (Garcin *et al.*, 1966; Weller, 1967; Thomas and Lascelles, 1967; Webster *et al.*, 1967; Dyck and Gomez, 1968).

Evidence of axonal degeneration is less frequently encountered than segmental demyelination. When it is seen, the axon shows a loss of neurofilaments and neurotubules with replacement of these elements by an amorphous granular material, and, occasionally, by membrane-bound glycogen granules.

The separation of the myelin lamellae and the degeneration of the tubular configuration of the sheaths described by Lampert and Schochet and by Schlaepfer resemble the changes induced by diphtheria toxin in experimental animals (Webster *et al.*, 1961; Weller, 1965; Allt and Cavanagh, 1969) or by X-irradiation (Massurovsky *et al.*, 1967) or spinal barbotage (Bunge *et al.*, 1960). The axonal changes, that is to say, the granular disintegration of the neurofilaments, is also seen in conditions other than lead poisoning, for example in the distal stumps of axotomized neurones (Vial, 1958; Honjin *et al.*, 1959; Wechsler and Hager, 1962) and in isoniazid (INH) neuropathy (Schlaepfer and Hager, 1964).

The relative paucity of axonal degeneration seen with the electron microscope may be indicative that the change in the myelin sheath is only a transient phenomenon, and that regeneration is sufficiently rapid to prevent gross deterioration in the structure of the axon. Schlaepfer (1968) considers this to be the case and that the accumulation of glycogen-like particles, which are also to be seen in INH neuropathy (Schlaepfer and Hager, 1964) and in tetanus toxin poisoning (Perocchia, 1966), may reflect a more chronic degeneration of the axon.

B. Neurophysiological Studies

There is no consistency in the results of neurophysiological investigations in lead poisoning. In human cases there is usually no significant decrease in mean maximum conduction velocity (MMCV) (Preiskel, 1958; Simpson *et al.*, 1964; Delwaide and Chantraine, 1965; Catton *et al.*, 1970) although contrary evidence has been presented by other workers (Sessa *et al.*, 1965; Seppäläinen and Hernberg, 1972). There is often, however, other evidence of defects in the peripheral nervous system, particularly abnormalities of the electromyogram (EMG) including the presence of fibrillation and polyphasic potentials suggesting some degree of denervation of the muscles (Hausmanowa-Petrusewicz *et al.*, 1962; Delwaide and Chantraine, 1965; Catton *et al.*, 1970). The disparity in these results is most likely due to there being different degrees of axonal damage in the patients being studied. So long as a proportion of the fastest conducting fibres is intact, the MMCV will be normal. Using a method which measures conduction in the slowest fibres (CVSF) in the ulnar nerve, Seppäläinen and Hernberg (1972) demonstrated subclinical effects in lead workers which were, however, unrelated to other parameters of lead absorption. Much earlier, Lane and Lewy (1935) had shown alterations in chronaxie in lead workers in the absence of neurological signs and they suggested that this investigation might form part of a screening procedure for men exposed to lead. Changes in chronaxie have also been observed in workers handling leaded petrol (Kiryakov, 1963).

In guinea pigs with lead poisoning, Fullerton (1966) was able to demonstrate alteration in MMCV in a proportion of animals, but baboons with experimental plumbism showed no such change, and indeed, no histological evidence of any neurological abnormality (Hopkins, 1970).

Experiments with the superior cervical ganglion of the cat have demonstrated that in concentrations of 5–40 μM/litre, lead produces a pre-synaptic block in neural transmission by reducing the release of acetylcholine. Post-ganglionic conduction was not affected. The addition of excess calcium reversed the pre-synaptic block in conduction and restored the output of acetylcholine (Kostial and Vouk, 1957).

Lead has also been shown to bind to the subneural part of the motor end plate following the injection of lead salts *in vivo* or immersing muscle preparations *in vitro* (Sávay and Csillik, 1958, 1959; Csillik, 1965). In the tibialis anterior of the rat the sites of lead binding are closely related to the sites of calcium release but distinct from sites of cholinesterase activity (Nakamura *et al.*, 1967).

These experiments suggest a means whereby lead may produce some of its effects on neural conduction through competitive interaction with calcium ions.

C. Lead Encephalopathy

Encephalopathy is an uncommon feature of lead poisoning in adults although it does seem to be a particular risk in America amongst drinkers of moonshine whisky (Whitfield *et al.*, 1972). In children with the disease encephalopathy is seen much more frequently. There are no features peculiar to lead encephalopathy (McKhann, 1932) and the diagnosis is arrived at by a positive history of exposure to lead and the finding of other indices of lead poisoning. Lateralizing signs may be present in about a third of cases (Whitfield *et al.*, 1972) but are not diagnostic. Papilloedema, retinal haemorrhages and optic atrophy are all reported complications of lead encephalopathy and lesions of all the cranial nerves have at one time or another been attributed to lead poisoning (Hay, 1950). Primary optic atrophy was reported commonly by early workers (up to 10 per cent of women exposed to lead by Prendergast (1910) for example) and many other authors wrote on the ocular changes in lead poisoning, including amblyopia, retinal oedema, retrobulbar neuritis, scotomata, cataracts and extra-ocular muscle paralysis (Loewe, 1906; Alexander, 1909; Williams, 1911; Brose, 1915; Sautter, 1922; Sherer, 1935). These changes are seldom referred to nowadays.

Changes in the cerebro-spinal fluid (CSF) are not pathognomonic except for an increase in lead content. Cantarow and Trumper (1944) found the concentration of lead in the CSF of persons with no exposure was in the range of 0·001–0·040 mg per cent, but that this value might be as high as 0·35 mg per cent in patients with encephalopathy. The CSF pressure is usually raised and in addition, the protein content may be elevated and there may be an increase in the number of white cells, either lymphocytes or polymorphs (Mosny and Malloizel, 1907; Hay, 1950; Hess, 1961; Crutcher, 1963; Morris *et al.*, 1964; Law and Nelson, 1968; Whitfield *et al.*, 1972). The main value of lumbar puncture lies in excluding other causes of encephalopathy. Brain scan and electroencephalograms are unhelpful in making the diagnosis (Whitfield *et al.*, 1972).

Histological examination of brains from fatal cases shows generalized perivascular monocytic and polymorphonuclear infiltration, especially around the small capillaries. Patchy areas of demyelination may occur and all stages of neuronal degeneration are seen with proliferation of glial tissue. Macroscopically the brains are swollen and oedematous with flattened convolutions and small haemorrhagic foci in the meninges (Akelaitis, 1941; Cumings, 1959; Popoff *et al.*, 1963, Whitfield *et al.*, 1972).

D. Lower Motor Neurone Lesions

Lower motor neurone lesions were described in association with chronic lead poisoning by Kinnear Wilson in 1907. He noted distal symmetrical wasting of the muscles with weakness and in some cases, involvement of the pyramidal tract. In Aran's original description of motor neurone disease (1850), three of his eleven cases had had contact with lead and two of these had exhibited frank plumbism, but he did not consider it of aetiological significance. Other authors since then have reported varying degrees of upper and lower motor neurone involvement associated with a history of contact with lead (Campbell, 1955; Simpson *et al.*, 1964; Livesley and Sissons, 1968; Campbell and Williams, 1968; Campbell *et al.*, 1970).

Whilst the classic syndrome of motor neurone disease (MND) may be found in patients with a good history of lead exposure, there is also a more benign clinical variant. This is characterized—apart from an exposure to lead—by a symmetrical weakness of predominantly lower motor neurone type and a slow progression (Campbell *et al.*, 1970).

The role of lead in producing symptoms of MND is not understood. In a detailed investigation of heavy metal metabolism in a series of 31 patients with MND, 9 of whom may have had exposure to lead, there was no increase in urinary lead excretion (Currier and Haerer, 1968). Similarly in their study of 74 patients with the disease, Campbell *et al.* (1970) were unable to show any increase in bone lead concentration as compared with a control group, despite the fact that 15 per cent of the patients gave a history of extensive lead exposure. These results do not rule out the possibility that exposure to lead in the past might initiate a process of degeneration in the lower motor neurone which is not clinically apparent until many years later and when there is no biochemical evidence of increased lead absorption. Campbell *et al.* (1970) consider that lead released from bone may be a factor in producing the disease, and it is interesting to compare the findings of Newton-John and Morgan (1968) that bone loss commences in man between the ages of forty-five and sixty-five with the peak incidence of MND of fifty-five.

Some improvement in symptomatology has been reported following treatment with chelating agents (Livesley and Sissons, 1968; Campbell *et al.*, 1970) which supports the role of lead in the production of the disease in some cases.

E. Aetiology

The agent responsible for causing the pathological lesions in the nervous system has not been identified. The obvious candidates, the haem precursors, have been investigated to this end. Purified PBG and porphyrins have been shown to be pharmacologically inactive (Goldberg *et al.*, 1954) and Weatherall (1954) in his authorative review of the effects of drugs on porphyrin metabolism concluded that there was little evidence to support the view that porphyrins had any significant pharmacological actions apart from photosensitization. ALA also has been reported to be without adverse pharmacological effects (Jarrett *et al.*, 1956) although recently McGillion and Goldberg (1973) have shown that it potentiates the action of noradrenaline. Gibson and Goldberg (1956) have suggested that some substance having PBG as a precursor might be essential in some way for the maintenance of normal myelin. A block in the synthesis of this hypothetical substance in the liver of patients with porphyria could lead to the excretion of excess PBG and ALA and at the same time cause demyelination (Goldberg, 1959). There is no further evidence to support this view, which would not, in any case, explain the lesion in lead poisoning since PBG is not excreted in excess in the urine.

Other speculations for the aetiology of the neuropathy of plumbism have been based on the possibility of direct or indirect effects of lead on vascular permeability. Popoff *et al.* (1963) studied five fatal cases of lead poisoning with encephalopathy. In three, histological examination of brain tissue showed perivascular oedema and petechial haemorrhages. In one chronic case, the veins showed some thickening with cellular disintegration of their walls. In view of their findings, Popoff *et al.* suggested that vascular damage was a major factor in the pathogenesis of the neurological disorder.

Experimentally, lead encephalopathy has been produced in suckling rats by feeding the mothers lead carbonate (Pentschew and Garro, 1966). When the brains of the affected animals were examined a striking proliferation of the endothelial cells of the capillaries was found. An interference with the blood–brain barrier was observed, and an abnormal permeability to Trypan blue and Thoratrast could be demonstrated even before changes became apparent with the light microscope (Lampert *et al.*, 1967). The way in which lead apparently interferes with the permeability of the capillaries of the brain is not clear but it may be as the result of an interference with some energy-regulating system which differentiates the blood–brain barrier capillaries from less-differentiated capillaries. This mechanism may also account for the transitory psychotic episodes of porphyria (Pentschew and Garro, 1966) and an increased vascular permeability might prevail in the capillaries of the peripheral nerves to account for the peripheral neuropathy. Lampert and Schochet (1968) noted the presence of abnormal vessels showing endothelial proliferation and found also that there were widened spaces between the nerve fibres of affected nerves suggestive of an accumulation of excess tissue fluid. The perineurium has been shown to be an effective barrier to the diffusion of macromolecules (Waggener *et al.*, 1965) and the exudation of protein-rich material from abnormally permeable vessels within the endoneural compartments might produce oedema and damage to the Schwann cells either directly by increasing the pressure upon them, or indirectly, by causing ischaemia. Prolonged or repetitive oedema resulting from an impairment of the blood–nerve barrier has been discussed as a possible cause for inducing hypertrophic neuropathies (Krücke, 1941).

Finally, Schlaepfer (1968) has made the suggestion that the neuropathy of lead poisoning might be caused by initial damage to the supporting cells of the nervous system. The capsular cells in the dorsal root ganglion show a proliferation and accumulation of dense bodies in their cytoplasm, which have the electron microscope appearance of a heavy metal. Schlaepfer considered that lead interferes with the metabolism of the capsular cells in the dorsal root ganglion and that this, in turn, causes a degeneration of associated neurones and their axons. If the metabolism of the capsular cells is impaired then it is likely that the ganglion cells would degenerate since tissue culture studies have shown that the viability of the ganglion cell is dependant on a capsular cell investment (Peterson and Murray, 1960; Shimizu, 1965). Sensory neurones associated with damaged capsular cells show alterations in the neurotubular system and a paucity of endoplasmic reticulum similar to the changes seen after neuronal injury (Andres, 1961, 1963; Parnese, 1963). Changes in the tubular system of the axon such as Schlaepfer (1968) described in animals with lead neuropathy might well alter the axonal transport of material from the cell body since such movements are dependent upon the integrity of the neurotubule (Gonatas and Robbins, 1965). If the endoplasmic reticulum of the neurone is diminished as a result of the damage done by lead to the capsular cell then this, together with the defective tubular system would result in a significant diminution both of material available for transport and the transportation of that which was available. It is likely that those parts of the axon furthest from the cell body would suffer most as the result of diminished axon flow, and this could explain the predominance of distal degeneration.

The combination of capsular degeneration and segmental demyelination may possibly reflect a common metabolic lesion affecting the supporting satellite cells of the dorsal root ganglion and the Schwann cells of the peripheral nervous system, and it is interesting to note that these two types of cell have a common embryological origin (Detwille and Kehoe, 1939). It is impossible to speculate what the metabolic lesion might be, particularly since the combination of capsular degeneration and demyelination is found in other diseases also, for example diabetic neuropathy (Greenbaum *et al.*, 1964; Thomas and Lascelles, 1966) and hypertrophic neuritis (Marie and Bertrand, 1918; Thomas and Lascelles, 1967).

V. THE KIDNEY

A. Acute Lesions

The effects of lead on the kidney have been the subject of much debate. During the latter part of the last century and the early years of the present century there was no hesitation in ascribing renal damage to the action of lead and a condition of nephropathia saturnina was in wide usage (Lancéreaux, 1881a, b; Leyden, 1883; Gayler, 1887; Legge and Goadby, 1912; Oliver, 1914; Volhard and Fahr, 1914; Ophlüs, 1915; Pejic, 1928). By the 1930s, however, and for several years after, many writers, particularly in America, were expressing doubts about renal lesions in plumbism (Mayers, 1927; Belknap, 1936; Dreeson *et al.*, 1941; Mayers, 1947; Humperdinck, 1948; Johnstone, 1948; Greenfield and Gray, 1950; Hunter, 1955). Nevertheless, ample evidence has now accumulated which firmly establishes that lead can cause renal damage. The classic description of these changes was presented by Blackman in 1936 and his findings have since been confirmed in human and animal studies (Sroczyński *et al.*, 1954, Cohen *et al.*, 1960; Radošević *et al.*, 1961; Hass *et al.*, 1964; Richet *et al.*, 1964; Dallenbach, 1964; Albahary *et al.*, 1965; Tange *et al.*, 1965; Totovic, 1965; Gallé and Morel-Maroger, 1965; Morgan *et al.*, 1966; Emerson, 1967).

The main structural changes seen in acute lead poisoning principally affect the proximal convoluted tubules. The epithelial cells in this region atrophy and then show signs of regeneration. There is an increase in the intertubular connective tissue, thickening of the tubular basement membrane and round-cell infiltration. The mitochrondria of the cells of the proximal tubules swell and degenerate. The glomeruli may show signs of increased cellularity and changes in the basement membrane of the glomerular capillaries and foot processes of the epithelial cells has also been reported (Cohen *et al.*, 1960).

The characteristic finding, however, is the presence of intranuclear inclusion bodies in the cells of the proximal tubule (Blackman, 1936; Wachstein, 1949; Morgan *et al.*, 1966; Goyer *et al.*, 1970). They are found in children and adults with lead poisoning, as well as in cases of poisoning in animals (Finner and Calvery, 1939; Dalldorf and Williams, 1945; Staples, 1955; Clegg and Rylands, 1966; Lock *et al.*, 1966, 1967). The inclusion bodies are eosinophilic in character and are best seen with the electron microscope which has demonstrated their presence in cells which appear normal with the light microscope (Beaver, 1961; Angevine *et al.*, 1962). They arise independently of the nucleolus and consist of a compact core surrounded by a loose filamentous periphery and scattered electron-dense particles. Occasionally there is a clear halo around the inclusion bodies (Figs 45 and 46).

The nature of the inclusion bodies has been investigated by a number of workers. It is generally agreed that they contain lead with detectable amounts of iron, calcium and glycogen (Phelan, 1959; Landing and Nakai, 1959; Goyer *et al.*, 1970). They appear to contain neither DNA nor RNA but they do contain a protein with a high content of —SH groups (Wolman, 1954; Richter *et al.*, 1968).

The origin of the protein associated with the intranuclear inclusions has yet to be established. It may be derived from pre-existing nucleoprotein or synthesized *de novo*, although most evidence favours the former view. For example, Müller and Stöcker (1964) were unable to detect the incorporation of ^{14}C labelled phenylalanine in inclusions found in the kidneys of rats with lead poisoning and Richter *et al.* (1968) proposed from their experiments that the inclusions resulted from the degradation and restructuring of a non-histone nucleoprotein. Choie and Richter (1972b), however, have produced some evidence that the protein may be synthesized in the cell cytoplasm, bound to lead and transported to the nucleus when it is polymerized into the characteristic fibrils. These authors have found cytoplasmic structures in association with the endoplasmic reticulum in the epithelial cells of the proximal tubule which they consider may be the precursors of the protein component of the intranuclear inclusion bodies. These authors have also noted that lead stimulates DNA synthesis in the rat kidney and raise the possibility of this being connected with the formation of the inclusion bodies (Choie and Richter, 1972a).

Inclusion bodies appear in the kidney before there is evidence of an increase in ALA excretion and it has been suggested that they may serve a protective role in accumulating soft tissue lead, thus minimizing toxic injury to other cytoplasmic organelles (Goyer *et al.*, 1970). This may be part of a general biological mechanism for protection against cellular damage by lead for similar inclusion bodies have also been found in the leaves of moss plants (Skaar *et al.*, 1973).

The number of inclusion bodies increases with increasing lead exposure (Goyer, 1968), and although it had been thought that they were not found until after a minimum of four weeks' exposure, recent work has indicated that they may be detected in rat kidneys within 24 hr of a single intraperitoneal dose of lead salts (Choie and Richter, 1972b). The

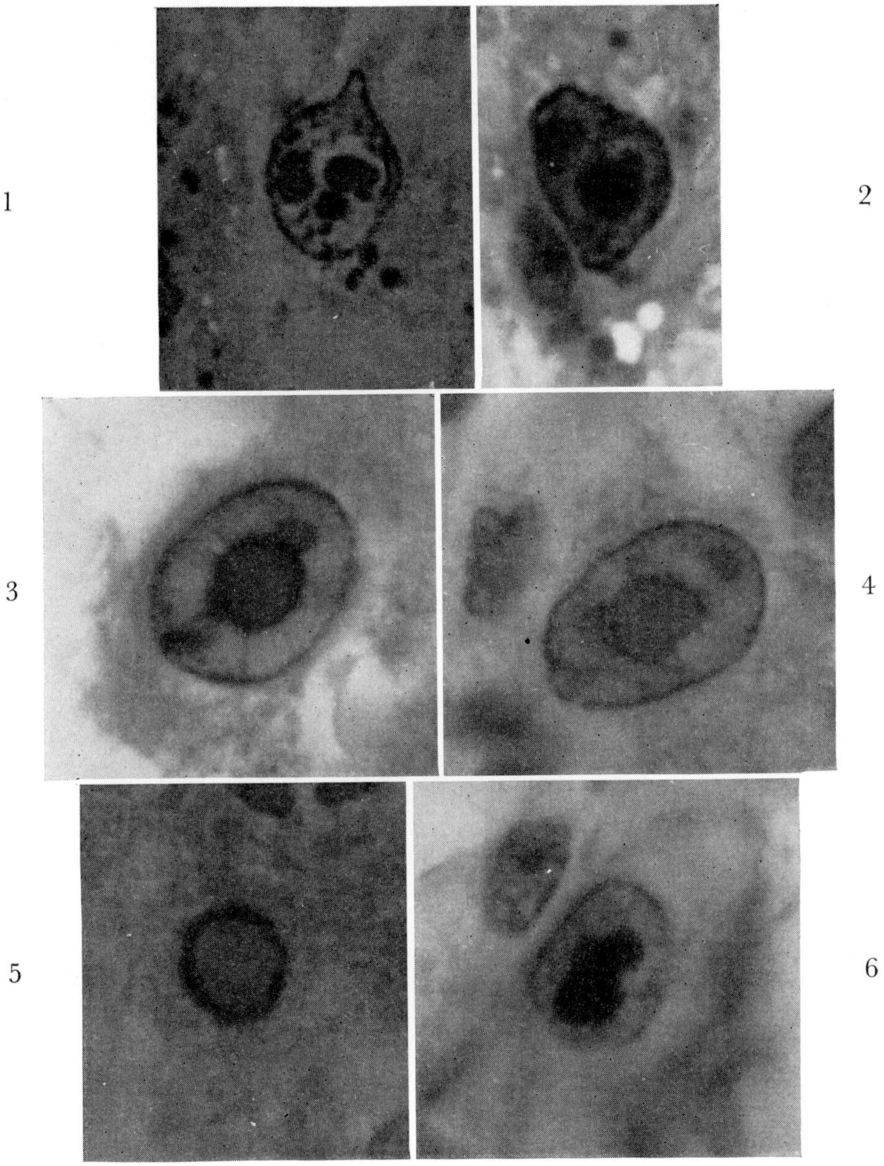

FIG. 45. 1. Nucleus of cell from proximal convoluted tubule of rat with experimental lead poisoning. Two inclusion bodies can be seen. The one at right has a core that took grey colour after staining with iron haematoxylin followed by toluidine blue. Dark body below two inclusions may represent clumped chromatin, ×2,500. 2. Intranuclear inclusion in cell of proximal tubule stained with basic fuchsin and toluidine blue. Inclusion body is intensely fuchsinophilic. Nucleolus is at left above inclusion, ×2,700. 3. Much enlarged nucleus in cell of proximal convoluted tubule. Two inclusions are attached to each other. Both have narrow Feulgen-positive rim. Chromatin is mainly situated at periphery of nucleus, ×2,300. 4. Two inclusions inside enlarged nucleus of cell of proximal tubule. Large inclusion body has a narrow, peripheral, Feulgen-positive rim. Feulgen-positive strands (? chromatin) radiate outwards from this rim, ×2,300. 5. Fast green stain for histones after extraction of nucleic acids with trichloroacetic acid. Inclusion body is unstained, ×2,300. 6. Mercuric bromphenol blue stain for proteins. Inclusion body deeply stained by contrast with lightly stained chromatin, ×2,300. Reproduced with permission from Richter *et al.* (1968).

A

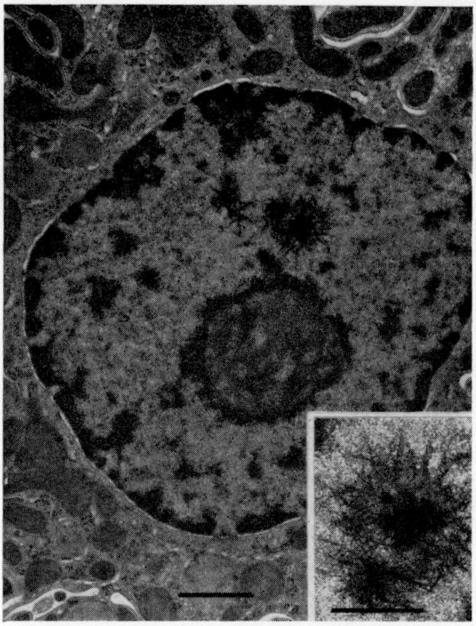

B

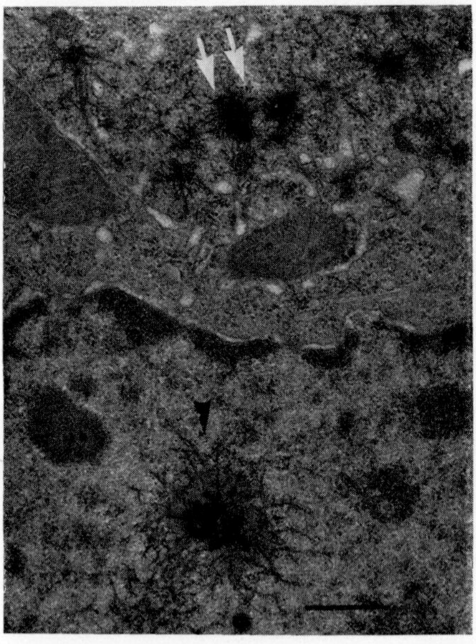

FIG. 46. A. EM of part of epithelial cell in proximal tublue of rat with experimental lead poisoning. Characteristic intranuclear inclusion body is seen above the nucleolus. Stained with uranyl acetate and Reynold's lead stain. Scale = 1 μm. Inset shows details of the inclusion body. B. EM of epithelial cell in proximal tubule of rat. A cytoplasmic structure (white arrow) is indicated in the location of the rough endoplasmic reticulum which resembles inclusion body (black arrow). Stained with uranyl acetate and Reynold's lead stain. Scale = 0·5 μm. Reproduced with permission from Choie and Richter (1972b).

dose of lead given in this experiment was large, however (0·05–0·20 mg/g body weight), and in all probability the production of these structures is a dose-related phenomenon.

Electron microscopy has also shown that the mitochondria of the proximal tubule cells are severely affected by lead both *in vivo* and *in vitro*, changes in rats appearing maximally about 10 weeks after exposure has begun (Goyer, 1968; Goyer *et al.*, 1968). The mitochondria become oval and rounded and the architecture of the christae is disordered. The disorganization is not specific to the kidney, similar changes having been described in mitochondria from liver cells (Banciu and Petrovici, 1968). The altered mitochondria in the kidney have a decreased rate of respiration and partially uncoupled oxidative phosphorylation and a proportion have impairment of electron transport (Goyer and Krall, 1969). After treatment with EDTA the structural changes may be partially reversed.

B. Acute Clinical Effects

The characteristic renal response to the lesions of acute lead poisoning is a Fanconi syndrome of aminoaciduria, glycosuria and phosphaturia (Emmerson, 1967). It is most commonly found in children but its occurrence in adults is well documented (Wilson *et al.*, 1953; Marsden and Wilson, 1955; Chisholm *et al.*, 1955; Cohen and Ahrens, 1959; Cohen *et al.*, 1960; Chisholm and Leahy, 1962; Crutcher, 1963). The full syndrome is only seen in the most severely affected cases and may be accompanied by renal rickets (Caffey, 1938; Follis *et al.*, 1943; Chisholm *et al.*, 1955). The pattern of aminoaciduria is similar to that found in other diseases characterized by the Fanconi syndrome, but the occurrence of fructose and citrate in the urine is unique to lead poisoning (Chisholm and Leahy, 1962).

The changes in renal function probably result from damage to the proximal tubule, either frank anatomical change or interference with transport mechanisms. In the latter context it is interesting that Thoelin *et al.* (1952) have noted a marked reduction in alkaline phosphatase activity in the cells of the proximal tubule in rats experimentally poisoned with lead. This may be an indication that more generalized enzyme inhibition occurs here as at other sites. Goyer (1968) has shown a positive correlation between kidney weight and the development of aminoaciduria in lead-poisoned rats. He suggested that, in addition to the tubular defect affecting aminoacid excretion, there may also be a transport defect for cations and water in the proximal tubule cells.

C. Sub-acute Effects

Renal function studies in lead workers have been undertaken and have been found abnormal in some cases. Crepet *et al.* (1956) and Rossi (1956) reported a reduction in renal plasma flow which they considered to be due to a vascular nephropathy. Radulescu *et al.* (1957) also noted impairment of renal function, as did Radošević *et al.* (1961), although in the experience of the latter authors, the changes were of a transient nature. Elevation of the urinary excretion of amino-nitrogen was found in 6 out of 24 workers exposed to lead fume or dust by Clarkson and Kench (1956). The relatively high proportion of men in this study showing renal tubular dysfunction indicates that renal lesions may occur more commonly than has been suspected. Lead also produces an adverse effect on the renin-aldosterone axis, presumably by damaging the cells of the juxta-glomerular apparatus. In a number of patients with lead poisoning there was no increase in plasma renin activity or aldosterone secretion rate in response to sodium deprivation (Sandstead *et al.*, 1970).

D. Chronic Nephropathy

Evidence that exposure to lead may produce a chronic nephropathy originates from early observations in Queensland. Between 1890 and 1930 lead poisoning in children was common because of the widespread use of lead paint on the exterior of houses (Gibson *et al.*, 1892; Breinl and Young, 1914; Nye, 1929). A concurrent increase in deaths from chronic nephritis was also noted at the time. Several lines of reasoning led to the conclusion that the two were causally related. Patients with so-called cryptogenic nephritis invariably gave a history of exposure to lead in childhood and had frequently suffered from clinical poisoning (Nye, 1929; McCann, 1932; Nye, 1933; Fairley, 1934; Murray, 1939; Henderson, 1954, 1955). In addition, the lead content of the bones of the skull was significantly higher in patients with cryptogenic nephritis than with other varieties of renal disease both in Queensland and in other parts of Australia (Henderson and Inglis, 1957; Henderson, 1958). This last work which indicated a higher exposure to lead amongst the group of patients with nephritis was confirmed by Emmerson (1963), who was able to show that these patients excreted significantly more lead in the urine in response to the EDTA provocation test than normal subjects or patients with other renal disease. Finally, a follow-up study of patients with childhood lead poisoning revealed that they had a much greater than expected incidence of chronic renal disease and its complications with a resultant increase in mortality (Henderson, 1954). Histologically, the kidneys show coarse granularity with gross cortical atropy and interstitial fibrosis. The number of glomeruli is reduced and there is hypertrophy of the tubules of the remaining nephrons (Emmerson, 1967).

The natural history of the disease varies considerably and is presumably dependent upon the degree of damage sustained. Many of Nye's patients died in their early twenties (Nye, 1933), but the prognosis is now improved. Henderson (1955) reported that the mean age of death of his patients was about forty, but Emmerson (1967) found that many patients were living to fifty and beyond.

The Australian experience has been confirmed elsewhere, although the incidence of subsequent renal damage is less than reported there. Tepper (1963), found that fewer than one per cent of persons having had lead poisoning twenty years previous to his study developed chronic nephropathy, but the difference is likely to be due to a difference in exposure. Amongst moonshine whisky drinkers chronic nephropathy is common (Morgan *et al.*, 1966; Sandstead *et al.*, 1970).

Chronic renal disease amongst workers exposed to lead seems to be less common than it was, reflecting the improvement which has occurred in working conditions over the century. When industrial hygiene was poor a high incidence of renal disease, hypertension and vascular disease was noted together with an increased death rate from cerebro vascular accidents (Olliver, 1862; Lancéreaux, 1881a, b; Oliver, 1891b; Legge and Goadby, 1912; Oliver, 1914; Vigdorchik, 1935; Lane, 1949; Henderson, 1958; Lane, 1964). More recent studies have indicated that these effects have largely been eliminated in industry (Malcolm, 1971).

Renal neoplasms have been produced in animals as the result of prolonged exposure (Zollinger, 1953; Boyland *et al.*, 1962) and also in wild rats exposed to lead fumes from burning refuse (Kilham *et al.*, 1962). Tange *et al.* (1965) have suggested that this may be the result of continued aberrant development of the giant cell-forms seen during the regeneration of the proximal tubular epithelium. There is, however, no increase in mortality from neoplasms amongst workers with known lead exposure (Dingwall-Fordyce and Lane, 1963).

E. Gout

Plasma uric acid levels are significantly higher in patients with lead nephropathy than in patients with comparable renal failure from other causes (Emmerson, 1963, 1965). The cause of the hyperuricaemia is due to a defect in the tubular secretion of uric acid (Emmerson, 1965; Ball and Sorensen, 1969) although Ludwig (1957) has proposed that it is due to an increased nucleoprotein turnover. Ball and Sorensen's detailed study of three patients with gout caused by drinking moonshine whisky demonstrated that three-quarters of the daily turnover of uric acid undergoes extrarenal elimination as compared with one-quarter to one-third in normal subjects. The rate of uric acid clearance is much more severely curtailed than either creatinine or inulin clearance. The finding that the healthy relatives of patients with saturnine gout also have a higher-than-normal incidence of hyperuricaemia, however, raises the question whether an inherited factor may be in some way responsible for the development of gout in patients with chronic lead nephropathy (Emerson, 1964).

The incidence of gout in lead poisoning is generally considered to be low, although more than 50 per cent of patients with chronic lead nephropathy may exhibit the disease. Ball and Sorensen (1969), however, found that 37 of the 43 admissions for gout to their hospital in 1967 were caused by drinking lead-contaminated liquor.

VI. EFFECTS ON OTHER ORGANS

A. The Thyroid

Patients with lead poisoning have been shown to have an impaired ^{131}I uptake by the thyroid, an effect which is responsive to thyroid-stimulating hormone (Sandstead *et al.*, 1966) and there have been cases of thyroid dysfunction presenting clinically in which lead has been suggested as an important aetiological factor (Porritt, 1931; Kremer and Martin, 1955).

Lead impairs the uptake of iodine in thyroid slices (Singerland, 1955) and its effect has been studied in experimental animals (Sandstead and Galloway, 1967). Rats receiving lead in their drinking water in a concentration of 8 or 12 mg/litre showed a decrease in ^{131}I uptake, conversion ratio and *in vitro* 24-hr ^{131}I uptake. The effects were of a lesser degree in males than in females. Sheep suffering from chronic lead poisoning also appear to have reduced thyroid activity judging from the low levels of protein-bound iodine in their serum (Soldatović *et al.*, 1966). Lead may act to depress thyroid function by inhibiting —SH groups or by displacing iodine in a protein sulphonyl iodine carrier (Sandstead and Galloway, 1967).

B. The Heart

Myocarditis has been noted as a concomitant symptom in children dying with lead encephalopathy (Kline, 1960), and Freeman (1965) reports a single case of a girl of three who recovered after treatment with EDTA.

There have also been isolated reports of abnormal ECG findings in adults with the disease. Read and Williams (1952) found inverted T-waves in the left chest leads in a male negro patient with depression of the conducting system and Myerson and Eisenhauer (1963) studied two patients both with first degree heart block, one of whom also showed ectopic atrial pacemakers. In both studies, the ECG reverted to normal after treatment of their lead poisoning.

T-wave flattening and S–T depression together with a shortened P–R interval, low-voltage QRS complexes and conduction defects were found in 66 per cent of a group of adults aged forty-six or over with chronic lead poisoning, a rate four times that of a control group (Kośmider and Petelenz, 1962), whereas a comparable study reported by Greenfield and Gray (1950) showed no abnormalities. Rabbits with experimental lead poisoning, however, do show T-wave and QRS changes, and degeneration and fibrosis of cardiac muscle can be demonstrated histologically (Kośmider and Sroczyński, 1961).

C. Miscellaneous Biochemical Effects

A large number of diverse biochemical abnormalities have been reported in association with lead absorption and lead poisoning in both animal and human subjects.

1. *Effects on Enzymes*

Lead may affect enzyme activity in one of two ways. It may either produce tissue damage and release tissue enzymes resulting in an increased activity in the serum, or it may directly inhibit enzymes, usually those having active —SH groups in their molecule, and so diminish their serum activity.

The transaminases, serum glutamic oxaloacetic and serum glutamic pyruvic transaminase (SGOT, SGPT) have been reported as having an increased activity in experimental animals (Kanner, 1965; Geleriu and Strauss, 1972; Strauss *et al.*, 1972) but in human cases both positive (Waldman and Borman, 1959; Brigatti *et al.*, 1962, Hanke, 1964) and negative (Casula *et al.*, 1959, Balbo and Marucci, 1962; Corsi and Galzigna, 1963; Waldron, 1964b) findings have been reported. These differences most likely reflect differences in exposure and hence varying degrees of tissue damage. Animal studies indicate that transaminase activity rapidly returns to normal after heavy exposure and fluctuation in activity may be very labile (Minden *et al.*, 1964).

Other enzymes studied include acid and alkaline phosphatases, catalase, cholinesterase and aldolase. The activity of alkaline phosphatase is usually diminished in the serum in lead-poisoned animals (Kośmider, 1953, 1963; Selariu and Milhăescu, 1957; Minden *et al.*, 1964), although normal or only slightly diminished activity is found in the cells of the blood (Biondi, 1955; Nunziante-Cesaro *et al.*, 1956). The enzyme activity in the liver may or may not be reduced (Thoelin *et al.*, 1952; Minden *et al.*, 1964). Kośmider (1963) found reduced serum levels in men exposed to lead and showed that in rabbits the decrease in activity of the enzyme was correlated to the dose of administered lead and to the appearance of coproporphyrin in the urine.

Acid phosphatase activity is unchanged in human lead poisoning (Nunziante-Cesaro *et al.*, 1956; Hanke, 1963) but abnormal tissue activity has been reported in experimental animals (Yagihara, 1960; Minden *et al.*, 1964).

Enhancement of aldolase activity has been observed in lead-exposed workers which correlated with urinary lead excretion (Yaverbaum, 1963) but this has not been confirmed by other workers (Casula *et al.*, 1959; Hanke, 1964). Similarly, although catalase activity has been reported as being increased in both sheep (Soldatović and Petrović, 1963) and rabbits (Sroczyński and Jonderko, 1963) other studies have shown no such change (Haeger-Aronsen, 1964).

There is no disagreement, however, that cholinesterase activity is decreased in men exposed to lead, in patients with lead poisoning (Ruźdig, 1950; Casula *et al.*, 1959,, 1960a,b; Skripnichenko, 1964) and in animals administered lead (Belli *et al.*, 1955; Soldatović and Petrović, 1963; Stanković and Mokranjac, 1964; Geleriu and Strauss, 1972; Strauss *et al.*, 1972). This effect is noted with organic and inorganic lead although greater inhibition is seen with organic lead (Stanković and Mokranjac, 1964).

Several other enzymes in addition to those mentioned have been less extensively studied and this work has been reviewed by Grazianni and Sessa (1952) and de Bruin (1971).

An important development is the application of histochemical techniques which are indicating that in a number of differing situations lead is capable of suppressing cellular oxidation-reduction reactions and of inhibiting active transport mechanisms involving ATP (Camba *et al.*, 1963; Jonek *et al.*, 1963, 1965; Sroczyński and Zajusz, 1966; Makashev and Verbolovich, 1967).

2. *Amino-acids and Proteins*

Aminoaciduria consequent upon the renal lesions caused by lead has been commented upon in an earlier section. In children excreting amino acids in the urine, plasma levels were reported as being normal (Wilson *et al.*, 1953) and increased urinary excretion with normal plasma concentration was also found in cases of industrial poisoning (Linari *et al.*, 1963). More recently, however, there is evidence that the plasma concentration of individual amino acids may alter during experimental and occupational lead exposure (Halaceva *et al.*, 1968; Boyadjiev *et al.*, 1968). Lead workers with no symptoms were found to have decreased concentrations of methionine, cysteine, alanine, leucine and glutamic acid in their plasma, and these levels correlated well with blood lead concentrations and with length of exposure.

Electrophoresis of plasma proteins has shown that the albumin–globulin ratio is decreased. A drop in albumin and an increase in globulin both contribute to the fall in the ratio. All the globulin components separated electrophoretically are increased, but the γ-globulin fraction seems subject to the greatest variability (Paparopoli, 1955; Granati *et al.*, 1956; Sroczyński and Pierkarski, 1959; Afonova, 1960; Cervetti and Casucci, 1960; Kolkovski and Rajceva, 1961; Muller *et al.*, 1962; Ambrosi, 1962; Gel'fon and Zorina, 1964; Kośmider and Petocka, 1967). There have been a few reports which have noted a decrease in all plasma protein components (Kapetonović *et al.*, 1960) or of the γ-globulin fraction (Plamieniak and Smolik, 1963; Aldanazarov *et al.*, 1963) but the evidence greatly favours the opposite view.

Nago (1959) studied the lead content of the various plasma protein fractions after electrophoretic separation and found that it was concentrated in the albumin and α_1-globulin fractions.

Protein synthesis *per se* is adversely affected by lead. At a concentration of 1·0 μM lead inhibits protein synthesis in rabbit reticulocytes (Borsook *et al.*, 1957). The mechanism through which this effect is produced is not clear. Lead causes disaggregation of polyribosomes in rabbit reticulocytes (Waxman and Rabinowitz, 1966) and it also brings about a decrease of amino acid acceptance by transfer RNA (Farkas *et al.*, 1972). In addition tRNA is inactivated and its ability to bind to ribosomes is diminished. This inhibition is more impaired than the ability of tRNA to accept amino-acids. None of these effects fully explains the inhibition of protein synthesis because the threshold concentration below which lead is inactive against tRNA is greater than that at which protein synthesis is impaired.

Abnormalities in protein synthesis may account for the defects in coagulation which have been observed in lead workers (Cataldi and Odaglia, 1958; Saita, 1960; Casula *et al.*, 1960b, Sroczyński and Kossmann, 1967). The usual defect is an increase in prothrombin time and a deficiency of factor VII. Prothrombin synthesis by the liver may be deficient (Saita, 1960) and the defects return to normal with the administration of vitamin K (Casula *et al.*, 1960b).

4 Sub-clinical Effects

I. A CAUSE FOR CONCERN?

There is little doubt that human activity has increased the mobilization of lead into the environment, particularly through the use of lead alkyls in petrol. As a result, many people have questioned whether this widespread dissemination of lead will produce harmful effects in the population at large. The suggestion is not that there will be endemics of frank clinical lead poisoning, but rather that the lead will exert a chronic effect, resulting in increased morbidity and mortality. Young children are considered to be particularly at risk because the neurotoxic effects of lead may bring about permanent damage to the developing central nervous system which, it is thought could result in mental retardation of behavioural abnormalities.

The risks associated with the use of TEL were brought to attention very soon after its introduction in America by a number of deaths amongst workers involved in its manufacture (Kehoe *et al.*, 1934). Neurological symptoms were notably prominent and the relatively large concentration of lead in the brains of fatal cases was described (Norris and Gettler, 1925). In 1925 Hamilton and her colleagues reviewed the experience with TEL and thought that there was a real danger of chronic lead poisoning associated with garage work and a possible danger to the public from the lead in street dust (Hamilton *et al.*, 1925). However, Kehoe *et al.* (1934) examined a large number of men exposed to TEL and found no evidence of lead absorption. They concluded their paper by stating that there was no reason to suppose that a danger to public health existed from the use or distribution of leaded petrol. Two years later the same authors reported on their findings amongst garage mechanics and petrol-pump attendants (Kehoe *et al.*, 1936). They reiterated their belief that there was no danger inherent in exposure to leaded petrol although they did find that prolonged exposure might give rise to an increase in urinary lead excretion. Lind (1936) reinforced this view from his study of persons with exposure to leaded petrol in Denmark.

B

In 1928 a committee was set up by the Ministry of Health to enquire into the possible dangers to health resulting from the use of leaded petrol. Their final report appeared in 1930 (Committee on Ethyl Petrol, 1930). They concurred with the reports from America that the use of leaded petrol was unlikely to increase the amount of lead in the atmosphere to the point where it would constitute a risk to health, even to those who might experience the greatest exposure, such as traffic policemen and drivers of motor vehicles. Good ventilation in garages was felt to be an adequate safeguard against the risk from spillage and they felt that the risk of absorbing TEL by contact of petrol with the skin was so slight as to be negligible. In view of this it was advised that legislation was not required to control the use of leaded petrol but the committee made one recommendation which was not put into effect. This was that cans and pumps should be labelled to indicate the presence of lead in the fuel and to warn the user to avoid spillage and not to use the fuel for other purposes than motor fuel.

After the introduction of TML as an antiknock Kehoe again investigated the potential hazards to those handling petrol containing this compound and was convinced that there was no hygienic reason against its use (Kehoe *et al.*, 1963).

There is no doubt, however, that under certain circumstances leaded petrol can be dangerous and even fatal. Workers using leaded petrol as a solvent in the manufacture of cheap rubber shoes have been found to have a considerable morbidity, and fatalities have occurred (Choi, 1963; *The Times*, 1968) and this has also been reported in men having long-term exposure to petrol containing TEL (Namba *et al.*, 1961). Severe psychiatric disturbances have also been reported in persons handling leaded petrol in confined spaces or who have been exposed to fumes after spillage (Kahan, 1950; Giraud *et al.*, 1959; Schlang, 1961). Law and Nelson (1968) have also documented a case of encephalopathy developing in a woman who was a chronic petrol sniffer. These case histories are an indication that the public at large, and especially those who handle leaded petrol in the course of their employment, should be made fully conversant with the hazards involved and advised on appropriate safety measures.

None of the early investigators considered the long-term effects of the use of lead alkyls in petrol and indeed some authorities deny that there is such a condition as chronic organic lead poisoning (Kehoe, 1964b; Barry and Turner, 1964). Nevertheless, there have been a number of cases in the literature describing chronic neurological symptoms which have been ascribed to long-term TEL exposure, in the absence of signs or symptoms of inorganic lead poisoning (Pomerantseva, 1950; Skripnichenko, 1955; Kiryakov, 1959; Gasto, 1959). Although the symptoms are in no way specific it seems justifiable, at the very least, to acknowledge the condition if only to underline the toxicity of the causative agent.

It is the chronic sub-clinical effects, rather than overt poisoning, which has prompted more recent writers to express their concern (Bersin, 1958; Fatzer, 1961, 1962; Patterson, 1965; Stöfen, 1966, 1968, 1969a, b, 1970; Lehnert, 1969; Danielson, 1969; Craig, 1970; Bryce-Smith, 1971a, b, c, 1972a, 1973; Hicks, 1972). Patterson (1965) considers that the average resident of the United States is being subjected to a chronic lead insult as the result of the increased lead flux in the environment. Bryce-Smith (1971a, b, c, 1972a) is more precise in his appraisal of the possible dangers and is concerned chiefly with behavioural effects. He gives particular emphasis to the dangers which increased absorption of lead might have on the development of the central nervous system in children, on mental health and on its relation to criminal behaviour. In this connection, he has pointed to the increased number of first admissions to mental hospitals or units and noted the rising trend, especially amongst the young.

He has also referred to work by Lob and Desbaumes (1971) who studied the blood and urine lead concentrations amongst two groups of inmates in separate gaols in Switzerland. Although the original authors did not comment on it, Bryce-Smith considered that the urinary lead levels were abnormally low in relation to the blood levels. This suggested to him that the high blood levels found in the prisoners might be a reflection of impaired renal function, with respect to lead, rather than abnormally high exposure.

The first reference to the possible connection between lead absorption and criminality, based on Soviet toxicology and behavioural changes noted amongst workers exposed to lead, was made by Stöfen (1969a, b). It was recommended that the total body burden of convicts should be studied in order to try and substantiate this hypothesis. In a later paper (Stöfen, 1971) further evidence was presented in support of this view.

The opposition to these views has come principally from those whose experience has been in industrial work and who have been unable to discover ill-effects in men working with lead except when accompanied by a rise in the blood lead concentration above eighty micrograms per cent (Johnstone, 1966; Haley, 1966; Williams, 1971). Haley states specifically that the average individual is in lead balance and is not adding to his body burden by accumulation, but this is inconsistent with the unequivocal rise in skeletal lead concentration with age (see Ch. 2). Williams (1971) objected to Bryce-Smith's suppositions on the grounds that first admissions to hospital are not a reliable index of disease prevalence in the community. Indeed, even if there is more mental illness diagnosed it may reflect a growing awareness on the part of physicians and less reluctance on the part of patients to accept a diagnosis of mental disease, rather than a true increase in incidence, but it must be pointed out that Bryce-Smith had, in fact, been careful to take these factors into account (Bryce-Smith, 1972a). In this discussion, however, industrial experience is not necessarily the most useful on which to base an argument. Those who propose that environmental lead levels may induce sub-clinical effects are not suggesting that classical lead poisoning is likely to result. Nor are they primarily concerned with the effects on adults, but on young children at a time when the central nervous system is most susceptible to injury. At the same time, however, this is not intended to preclude the possibility that lead in doses which are insufficient to produce clinical signs may produce adverse psychological effects in adults as has been shown in the case of carbon disulphide (Hänninen, 1971). Indeed, reference has already been made to unpublished work on lead workers in which Hänninen has claimed that such *is* the case (Bryce-Smith, 1972a; *Lancet*, 1973).

Considerations other than those of health have also been raised against the suggestion that lead should be removed from petrol.

It is claimed that cars run on lead-free petrol emit an increased concentration of aldehydes, phenols and polynuclear hydrocarbons in the exhaust gas. The photochemical reactivity of the exhaust gas is also said to be increased, tending to greater smog formation (Felt and Kerley, 1971). In addition, it is stated that the investment costs to the oil companies in installing new plant to change refining techniques to those necessary for producing high-octane lead-free petrol are likely to result in a rise in petrol prices (Tims, 1971). Fuel consumption may be up to ten per cent greater using lead-free petrol (Myers, 1971). Engine wear, and especially valve wear, is said to be greater in a car run on lead-free petrol, so the overall cost to the motorist in deleading petrol may be considerable (Boddy, 1972). Not all these supposed ill-effects consequent upon removing lead from petrol will stand up to critical examination, however. If petrols of the same aromatic content are compared, then lead-free fuel has a *lower* emission of unburned hydrocarbons, although carbon monoxide emissions are largely unchanged. Again, lead additives far from protecting the engine, may increase engine wear (Civil Aviation Authority, 1972). Ethylene dichloride added as a lead scavenger produces hydrochloric acid as a by-product during combustion and this is responsible for a major part of the corrosion of some engine components including silencers and piston rings, and for the deterioration of lubricating oils. The wearing of valve seats only occurs with certain engine designs and then only under extreme conditions when the engine is run for prolonged periods at abnormally high revs. It is easily prevented by a phosphate additive of much lower toxicity than TEL or by a minor modification of engine design.

With existing refining techniques, high-octane lead-free petrol may be produced readily and the cost would not be more than perhaps 1p a gallon. It is likely that the reduced maintenance which would be needed with lead-free petrol would offset the increase in petrol costs to the motorist. To some extent, however, these considerations have all been pre-empted by American legislation governing the quality of exhaust gases. One method of achieving the standards proposed is by the use of catalytic converters, but the activity of these catalysts is so severely affected by lead (Sorensen and Nobe, 1972) that their use would be completely uneconomical with lead present in petrol.

II. EVIDENCE FOR INCREASED LEAD ABSORPTION IN HIGH RISK GROUPS

Before considering ill effects caused by environmental lead, it is necessary to determine whether or not there is any evidence that persons in high-risk groups show an increased absorption. Two such groups suggest themselves. Firstly, urban communities, because they have a higher ambient lead level than those living in the country, and, secondly, children, because of their peculiar risks of exposure.

A. Lead Absorption in Urban Communities

Hofreuter *et al.* (1961) studied the blood lead concentration of groups ot people from six American cities and compared them with those of a rural population. Differences were found from one city to another, but the mean concentration of all the urban blood samples was 20 μg/100 g compared with the rural mean of 14 μg/100 g. This difference was highly significant, p $<$ 0·01 (Table 37). In Los Angeles, Thomas *et al.* (1967) also found a difference between the blood lead of those living in the city compared with people living on the coast. They were studying in particular, persons living near the freeway and the mean blood lead concentration for men in this group was 22·7 μg/100 g($n = 15$) whilst the mean of those living away from the freeway was 16 μg/100 g($n = 20$). Again there was a significant difference between the two means, $p < 0{\cdot}006$. There was no gradient from the freeway and it was not

Table 37

Blood lead concentrations in urban and rural communities

Site	n	Blood lead concentration $\mu g/100$ g Mean (SD)	
New Orleans	130	22	(9)
Dallas	128	18	(7)
Denver	131	19	(7)
Chicago	97	20	(8)
New York	112	20	(8)
Cincinnati	137	20	(8)
Rural	162	14	(6)

From Hofreuter *et al.* (1961)

considered that the higher blood leads in the group living near the freeway resulted directly from the exhaust emissions of passing cars.

Conversely, however, Daines *et al.* (1972) found that the blood lead concentration of female black subjects was a function of the distance they lived from a road which supported heavy traffic. For a group living 3·7 m from the road the mean blood lead concentration was 23·1 $\mu g/100$ g whereas from two other groups living 38·1 and 121·9 m from the road the means were 17·4 and 17·6 $\mu g/100$ g respectively.

In a recent study of blood lead levels in some London taxi drivers, Jones *et al.* (1972) found the mean concentration to be 28·7 $\mu g/100$ ml. They did not study a control group, instead they compared the concentrations in day-time and night-time drivers, finding no difference, although there was a significant difference in the carboxyhaemoglobin level from which they inferred greater exposure to exhaust fumes, even allowing for smoking habits. This investigation was criticised on a number of counts (Howard, 1972; Goldsmith, 1972; Bryce-Smith, 1972b) and without adequate controls it is difficult to know how to evaluate the results which the authors felt lay within the range of typical urban values.

Goldsmith and Hexter (1967) consider that there is a direct relationship between atmospheric exposure to lead and the blood lead concentration and that one can be predicted from the other (Fig. 47). Their regression line has been calculated from epidemiological data although they claim that reported experimental data fit well around the slope of their graph. Their equation for predicting blood lead concentrations from atmospheric levels has the form

$$\log_{10} \text{blood lead} = 1{\cdot}265 + 0{\cdot}2433 \log_{10} \text{atmospheric lead concentration.}$$

This work has been criticized by Kehoe (1968) principally because gastrointestinal absorption, which accounts for the larger part of an individual's exposure, was ignored, and also because such a relationship assumes a constant environmental lead concentration. In defending their position Goldsmith and Hexter (1968) point to the fact that the ratio of

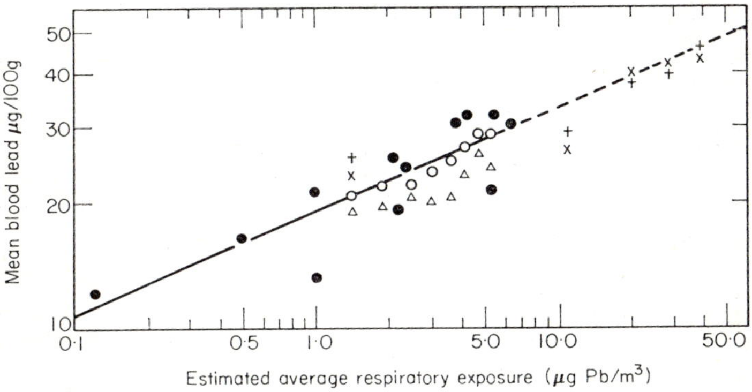

FIG. 47. Mean blood lead concentrations from epidemiological and experimental respiratory experiments. The regression line is constructed from epidemiological data only: ●, epidemiological data; ×, +, ○, △, experimental subjects. Reproduced with permission from Goldsmith and Hexter (1967).

lead absorption from the lungs is far greater than from the gut so that even though more lead is presented to the gut than the lungs, the amounts absorbed are roughly equal. A more serious criticism is that the data used were the results of blood lead and air lead estimations which were performed on samples collected at different times. Constructing a regression line using blood and air lead analyses collected at the same time and place gives only weak positive correlation ($r = 0{\cdot}22$) (Goldwater, 1972). Nevertheless, Goldsmith and Hexter are able to show that results predicted from their model give a close fit to observed values and this holds for the study done on London taxi drivers (Goldsmith, 1972).

The relationship which Goldsmith and Hexter have derived indicates that blood lead concentration will increase as a function of atmospheric lead exposure. Comparing blood lead concentrations between two groups can be misleading, however, if the composition of the groups is not defined specifically. Thus, females have lower blood leads than males, so that an imbalance in the sex ratios can bias the results. Smoking habits also affect blood lead concentration. Lead arsenate is still widely used as an insecticide on tobacco plants and although most of the lead remains in the ash and tar (Conway, 1940), Cogbill and Hobbs (1957) showed that with some cigarettes up to 0·3 μg of lead could be taken in with each inhalation. Smoking habits should therefore be identical in groups under comparison so as not to influence the result.

Hofreuter and his colleagues (1961) took all these factors into account and were able to show that for each sub-group, urban lead concentrations were in excess of rural values.

Hair lead estimations have also been shown to be higher in city dwellers than in those living in the country (Tonomura *et al.*, 1965; Hammer *et al.*, 1971) whilst within cities, traffic policemen have a higher than average lead content in their hair indicating heavy exposure (Speizer *et al.*, 1972).

Present-day exposure to lead, however, may be less than it was a century ago, at least in America, judging from a survey conducted by Weiss and his colleagues (Weiss, 1972; Weiss *et al.*, 1972). They obtained samples of hair dating from 1870–1923 and found it contained a significantly higher lead concentration than modern hair from persons with no known industrial exposure. The authors considered that dietary lead exposure might have been greater a century ago due to the extensive use of glazed earthenware and that this factor accounted for the marked difference in lead content (Table 38).

Table 38

	Lead in hair, μg/g dry weight Mean (SD)				
	n	1870–1923	*n*	Contemporary	*p*
Adults	36	164·24 (20·7)	119	16·23 (0·97)	<0·01
Children	20	93·36 (16·3)	28	6·55 (1·17)	<0·01

From Weiss *et al.* (1972)

To establish whether body burden of lead correlates with the length of time spent in a city, Nusbaum *et al.* (1965) analysed specimens of rib and calvarium obtained from autopsies carried out at Los Angeles County Hospital. Sex differences were noted and a difference was noted between smokers and non-smokers (Table 39). There was no correlation, however, between bone lead concentrations and length of stay in the area.

Table 39

Sex differences and the effect of smoking on bone lead concentration (Bone lead concentration mg/100 g dry wt.) Mean (SD)

	Smokers			Non-smokers		
	n	Calvarium	Rib	*n*	Calvarium	Rib
Males	23[a]	76 (5)	84 (5)	9	59 (4)	66 (7)
Females	15	63 (5)	59 (4)	23	58 (4)	63 (4)

[a] $n = 24$ for rib
From Nusbaum *et al.* (1965)

B. Lead Absorption in Urban Children

In children, ingestion is a more important route for lead absorption than inhalation because of their habits of exploring their environment through their mouth. Pica is a habit most children develop and its association with lead poisoning was first postulated by Ruddock (1924). In the great American cities children in the slum areas are especially prone to develop lead poisoning from eating flakes of paint. A large number of surveys have been reported from cities in America including Baltimore, Chicago, Cincinnatti, Cleveland, New York, Norfolk and Washington (Bradley et *al.*, 1956; McLaughlin, 1956; Cohen and Ahrens, 1959; Ingalls *et al.*, 1961; Christian *et al.*, 1964; Griggs *et al.*, 1964; Blanksma *et al.*, 1969; Guinee, 1971; Challop *et al.*, 1972). In several cities epidemiological surveys of blood lead concentrations in children at risk have revealed large numbers with markedly elevated levels. Lin-Fu (1972) has summarized a great deal of the recent data and this is shown in Table 40. At least a fifth of all the measurements are in excess of 40 μg of lead/100 ml and in terms of absolute numbers the situation is extremely grave. When screening programmes are regularly employed, there is a tendency for the number of high values to fall. This is because in the first instance the survey measures the prevalence of high blood leads amongst the population, whereas later, an incidence rate is determined (Guinee, 1972).

Hair lead surveys amongst children at risk have confirmed their excessive lead exposure (Pueschel *et al.*, 1972). Of 705 children screened in

Table 40

Blood lead concentration in urban children

City	Years of study	n	Blood lead concentration μg/100 ml % of children >40	>50	>60	>70	>80
Baltimore	1968–1970	2,350	28·2				
Chicago	1967–1970	120,000	20	4			
Washington	1970–1971	1,158	22	12			2·2
New Haven	1969–1970	1,897	29·8		9·5		
Newark	1970	594	38·9		9·5		
New York	1970	84,493	28·7		5·9	2·2	
Philadelphia	1970	3,496	32·3		14·9		

Based on Lin-Fu (1972)

Boston, 98 were considered to require active treatment. The mean hair lead concentration in the group was 118 μg/g (SD 100).

III. THE EVIDENCE FOR HARMFUL EFFECTS OF CURRENT ENVIRONMENTAL LEAD LEVELS

The concept that there is a threshold below which lead is metabolically inert, and particularly that there is a range of safe blood lead concentrations has been challenged in recent years (*Lancet*, 1973). Studies of ALA-d activity have shown unequivocally that present-day levels of environmental contamination are sufficient to produce inhibition of this enzyme (Hernberg and Nikkanen, 1970). In persons with no industrial exposure and who were clinically well, there was a direct negative correlation between blood lead concentration and ALA-d activity (Fig. 48). Inhibition of the enzyme is the most sensitive index of lead exposure and in men newly engaged in lead work, a measurable decrease in activity is noted in the first few days (Hernberg *et al.*, 1972). Not only does contact with lead produce rapid inhibition of ALA-d but the effects are observed even when occupational exposure has long been discontinued. A group of men who had been in lead industries but who had discontinued this work for between three and seventeen years showed a lowered activity of ALA-d as compared with a control group (47·44 units/ml compared to 116·54 units/ml for the controls). This indicated that the lead absorbed during the years of exposure was still metabolically active (Přerovská and Teisinger, 1970).

Beattie *et al.* (1972b) found a negative correlation between blood lead concentration and ALA-d activity in a group of people living in houses in Glasgow supplied with water via lead pipes. The ALA-d activity also had a significant negative correlation with the lead content of the household water, the mean content of which was three and a-half times greater than the upper safe limit of 100 μg/l proposed by the World Health Organization (1971). None of those examined had signs of clinical lead poisoning but leaded domestic water was the cause of symptoms in

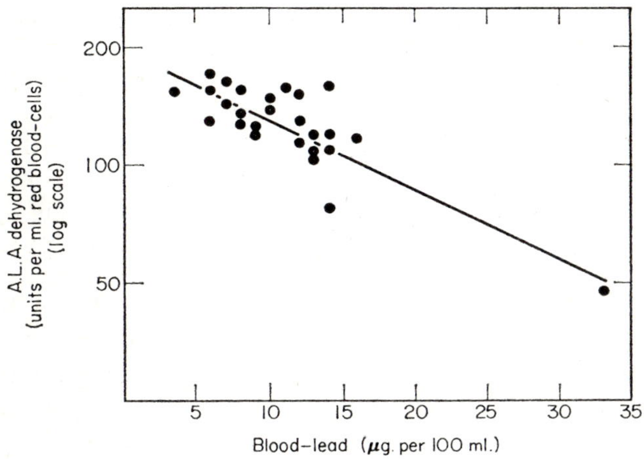

FIG. 48. Relationship between blood lead concentration and red cell ALA-d activity in 26 persons with no industrial exposure to lead. Reproduced with permission from Hernberg and Nikkanen (1970).

another group living in rural Scotland (Beattie *et al.*, 1972a). Nine of the fourteen persons examined had clinical or biochemical evidence of lead poisoning but in only one was the blood lead concentration greater than 80 μg/100 ml.

The question, whether environmental lead levels are likely to have any long-term effects, can be considered by examining whether there is any evidence of permanent damage in children, by considering the effects of sub-lethal doses in animals and by surveying the epidemiological evidence that lead is associated with other diseases.

A. Effects in Children

It is an old observation that lead is an abortifacient and female lead workers had a high rate of miscarriage. In a series of 123 studied by Paul (1860) there were 73 foetal deaths and into the twentieth century the abortion and still-birth rate was estimated at between 17 and 60 per cent (Aub *et al.*, 1925; Cantarow and Trumper, 1944). Women often resorted to using lead to rid themselves of unwanted pregnancies and many cases of lead poisoning were reported from this practice (Hall, 1905; Hall and Ransom, 1906). The very low birth rate in Dewsbury at the beginning the century was blamed on early abortion caused by the high lead content of the local water (Wynne, 1911). Recently it has been suggested that the high infant mortality rate in soft-water areas may be a consequence of the increase in lead content which is found in inverse relation to the calcium concentration (Crawford *et al.*, 1972).

The ability of lead to cross the placental barrier was inferred from its efficacy at procuring abortion and demonstrated many years ago (Oliver, 1891a, 1902, 1911; Bell, 1924; Aub *et al.*, 1925; Hamilton, 1929; Hansmann and Perry, 1940; Cantarow and Trumper, 1944). Cord blood has been shown to contain lead in concentrations approximating those found in maternal blood (Scanlon, 1971; Harris and Holley, 1972; Rajegowda *et al.*, 1972). There is a significant correlation between the two concentrations and the lower concentrations found in cord blood may be an indication that the foetal tissues are removing lead from the maternal blood at a rate faster than it can be replaced (Barltrop, 1969). The blood of newborns contains lead in concentrations similar to that in cord blood (Robinson *et al.*, 1958; Cubasik and Volasin, 1972).

It has been noted that the foetus is most susceptible to the effects of lead during the phase of rapid growth and it has been postulated that foetal tissues may be able to concentrate lead at least during the first sixteen weeks of gestation (Karlog and Møller, 1958).

In this context the high levels of lead found in the brains of stillborn infants (Table 30) are of considerable importance since they may well reflect generally high levels in the nervous system. Whether lead in the concentration found has any adverse effect on the developing central nervous system awaits investigation; but if it has, it is not possible to infer this retrospectively because the concentration of lead in the adult brain is *less* than in the infant as a comparison of the data in Tables 29 and 30 shows.

There have been reports that lead is teratogenic in some species. Anomalies in the tail and sacrum of foetal hamsters have been induced by feeding the mother lead (Ferm and Carpenter, 1967), an effect which is enhanced in the presence of cadmium (Ferm, 1969), whilst chick embryos seem to be particularly susceptible to the effects of lead. The characteristic lesion in chicks seems to be the development of hydrocephalus and meningocoeles (Butt *et al.*, 1952; Taylor and Carmichael,

1953; McLaughlin *et al.*, 1963) but in addition brain necrosis has also been induced (Karnofsky and Ridgway, 1952) as has cranioschisis (Butt *et al.*, 1952). There is no evidence that lead is teratogenic to humans and it has not been possible to produce developmental abnormalities in either the sheep or the cow (James *et al.*, 1966; Shupe *et al.*, 1967).

Although the abortifacient capacity which lead has may be the result of a direct effect on the foetus, pathological effects on the placenta could also play a role. Trophoblastic necrosis and placental haemorrhages have been attributed to lead (Baker, 1960) and it has also been shown to affect placental metabolism (Dawson *et al.*, 1965). Succinic dehydrogenase is inhibited in normal and toxaemic placentae, although to a much greater degree in the latter. Cytochrome oxidase is also severely inhibited in toxaemic placentae but the effect of lead on normal placentae is to increase the activity of this enzyme. Thus it seems that lead may severely depress oxidative metabolism in toxaemic placentae and make the continued existence of the foetus even more precarious.

The teratogenic effect awaits complete elucidation. Lead fed to rats in high doses (one per cent of the diet) has been shown to induce chromosomal aberrations in leucocyte cultures. The effects mainly involved single chromatids which suggested that the damage had occurred after the phase of DNA synthesis in the cell cycle (Muro and Goyer, 1969), although the effect could have been produced from an activation of DNA-ase. There is presumptive evidence that lead can enhance the activity of this enzyme from the finding of a marked increase in its urinary excretion in lead-poisoned rats (Krigman *et al.*, 1968). It remains to be seen if lead at lower doses can produce chromosomal damage before this mechanism can be blamed for embryonic defects.

Paternal factors have long been known to be significant (Oliver, 1891a, 1902, 1911; Tredgold, 1947). One recent well-documented case reports the birth of children with lethal malformations to a woman who had had normal deliveries previously. Her husband was diagnosed as having lead poisoning and after he had received treatment she produced normal children again, suggesting that his illness may have been causative (Van Assen, 1958). The findings of Egorova *et al.* (1966) and Golubovich *et al.* (1968) are of interest in this context, for they were able to show abnormalities in sperm morphology and motility together with alteration in chromosome division in animals given lead in doses which produced no other demonstrable effects.

It is well known that children who develop lead poisoning are liable to be left with permanent neurological damage, particularly if they had encephalopathy (McKhann, 1932; McKhann and Vogt, 1933; Levinson and Zeldes, 1939; Byers and Lord, 1943; Giannattasio *et al.*, 1952; Gibb and MacMahon, 1955; Mellins and Jenkins, 1955; Thurston *et al.*, 1955; Chisholm and Harrison, 1956; McLaughlin, 1956; Jenkins and Mellins, 1957; Bradley and Baumgartner, 1958; Byers, 1959; Cohen and Ahrens, 1959; White and Fowler, 1960; Smith *et al.*, 1963; Smith, 1964; Woods and Walters, 1964; Chisholm, 1965; Hardy, 1966; Perlstein and Attala, 1966; Lin-Fu, 1967; Weiner, 1970; Graef *et al.*, 1971). The damage may present as a gross anatomical lesion, Vogt (1932), for example, describing a ventriculogram showing internal hydrocephalus in a child of four who had had lead encephalopathy two years previously, or it may show itself as severe mental deficiency in a child who had progressed normally before contracting the disease (Berg and Zappella, 1964). Most often, however, follow-up studies have shown that the chronic effects are manifested through the children not doing as well at school as their peers, having a short attention span and being easily distracted. These effects constitute part of what is called the hyperactivity syndrome which may include more severe behavioural disturbances than those mentioned here.

Estimates of the percentage of children left with permanent damage vary. In the large series of Perlstein and Attala (1966) 39 per cent of children were left with permanent neurological sequelae, and this figure increased to 82 per cent in those who had encephalopathy. If children who have once had encephalopathy are subsequently re-exposed to lead, then they are invariably left with permanent damage (Chisholm and Harrison, 1956).

Neurological defects and failure to thrive were observed in a ten-week-old infant whose mother drank moonshine whisky and who had lead poisoning during pregnancy (Palmisano *et al.*, 1969) but treatment of lead poisoning with EDTA during pregnancy may spare the foetus (Angle and McIntyre, 1964).

Asymptomatic children may also have psychological or neurological impairment. Pueschel *et al.* (1972) followed-up a series of children who were found to have an increased body burden of lead on routine screening and were able to detect neurological and motor impairment in over a quarter of the forty-two traced after one-and-a-half years. There was an improvement in I.Q., however, and the children generally performed better during psychological testing than during the first examination.

Deficiencies in fine-motor adaptive and language functions were noted in children in low socio-economic groups in New Haven as compared with the Denver sample of children used to create the Denver Developmental Screening Test (Kotok, 1972). The New Haven children were divided into two groups with blood lead concentrations greater or less than 60 μg per cent. Within these two groups no differences in develop-

lead levels as a cause of hyperactivity. If they had assumed that the levels could have been higher or lower, and used a two-tailed t-test, then the difference between the results of the blood lead concentration in the experimental group and the controls has a significance of 2·5–5 per cent compared with <1 per cent using the one-tailed t-test (Bulpitt, 1972).

The uncertainty as to whether lead ingestion is a precipitating or an aggravating factor in mental retardation still provokes considerable discussion and has not been resolved to the satisfaction of all the interested parties. Animal experimentation has shown that lead alkyls can inhibit glucose metabolism in brain slices. This is true of triethyl lead, diethyl lead and trimethyl lead (Cremer, 1959, 1962a; Aldridge *et al.*, 1962). It has been claimed that TEL acts to inhibit brain metabolism in rats *in vivo* (Vardanis and Quastel, 1961) but attempts to repeat these experiments did not yield the same results (Cremer, 1962b). In rabbits TEL has been shown to inhibit monoamine oxidase activity (Galzigna *et al.*, 1964) and a build up of serotonin has been found in brain homogenates incubated with TEL (Magistretti *et al.*, 1961).

Inorganic lead was shown to inhibit glucose metabolism in brain slices by Dolowitz *et al.* (1937) but later work failed to confirm this observation (Cremer, 1959). Nevertheless, suckling rats have been shown to have an 80–90 per cent reduction in the activity of ALA-d in the brain when their mothers are fed with lead (Millar *et al.*, 1970).

The evidence is sufficient to indicate that organic and inorganic lead can produce disturbances in brain metabolism. It is certain that it can produce lasting mental impairment and so it would seem desirable that every effort be made to reduce the body burden of children to as low a level as possible.

B. Sub-clinical Effects in Animals

Following administration of organic lead, animals become excitable especially in their reaction to sudden noise and movement (Cremer, 1959; Castellino *et al.*, 1963) but the ability of rats to perform standard psychological tests is not affected. High doses of TEL do not significantly impair learning or memory even in the presence of toxic symptoms (Bullock *et al.*, 1966). Lead acetate has also been reported to be without effect on learning and memory in rats (Brown *et al.*, 1971). Gusev (1960), however, has shown that changes in the patterns of conditioned reflex behaviour occur in animals exposed to low concentrations of atmospheric lead. This was also noted in goldfish when sublethal doses of lead (as lead nitrate) were added to the water in their tanks (Weir and Hine, 1970). In terms of concentration mercury was more potent than lead, but in terms of fractions of the lethal concentration the converse was true. Thus, the lowest concentration of lead which impaired performance was 0·07 ppm and of mercury 0·003 ppm. These represented 1/1570 of the LC_{50} and 1/857 of the LC_1 for lead and 1/273 of the LC_{50} and 1/120 of the LC_1 for mercury (Weir and Hine, 1970).

In terms of affecting mortality, claims have been made that in concentrations approximating to those in typical human tissues lead produces an increased mortality rate in male (but not female) mice, and of both male and female rats (Schroeder *et al.*, 1963a, b, 1965). Male rats did not show an excess of deaths until they were more than eighteen months old, whereas females showed a steady increase in mortality from six months. Growth was not adversely affected in either species. No pathological effects were observed to account for the increased mortality and it was found unexpectedly that the incidence of tumours was significantly less in male mice and both male and female rats than in the controls (Schroeder *et al.*, 1964, 1965).

In these early experiments both species were deficient in trivalent chromium which appears to be an essential trace element for these animals (Schwartz and Mertz, 1959; Mertz *et al.*, 1961, 1965). The control animals in all cases were probably also deficient in chromium and so comparison should have been correctly made with animals receiving chromium. There is a possibility that in the absence of chromium, lead has an enhanced effect, and some support for this idea is given in later experiments when it was found that with adequate supplies of chromium, lead had no effect in increasing mortality (Schroeder *et al.*, 1970).

The harmful effects on reproduction of rats and mice in the presence of adequate chromium, however, has been demonstrated convincingly (Schroeder and Mitchener, 1971). Breeding animals were given drinking water containing lead in a concentration of 25 ppm. Mice on this regime produced fewer litters than controls and there was a considerable increase in runts and early deaths. The effects were so severe that by the second generation there were insufficient animals to carry on the experiment. In rats the effects were similar in that litter size was reduced and runting and early death common, but they were not so severe and litters were produced to the F_3 generation. The experiment showed that lead (and certain other trace elements) was incompatible with normal reproduction in doses which did not interfere with growth or individual survival.

Another sub-clinical effect which has been noted is the ability of lead to increase susceptibility to infection. In both rats (Selye *et al.*, 1961) and chicks (Truscott, 1970) lead has been shown to diminish resistance to bacterial endotoxins and in rats and primates it may even cause a massive sensitization to these agents (Di Luzzio, 1972). Mice infected with a strain of *Salmonella typhimurium* of limited pathogenicity were markedly more susceptible after intraperitoneal injection of lead nitrate. In the lead-treated animals there was a tenfold difference in the LD_{50} although none of them showed signs of lead poisoning (Hemphill *et al.*, 1971). Rats can also be rendered more susceptible to salmonella infection by the administration of TEL (Schroeder *et al.*, 1972). This diminished resistance might result either from the lead binding with antibodies (Williams *et al.*, 1954) or by an interference with the phagocytic activity of polymorphonuclear leucocytes (Rakkimova, 1968).

It is also of interest to note that inhalation by rats of a lead aerosol (particle size $<0{\cdot}1\ \mu$) reduced the number of alveolar macrophages in pulmonary washings although producing no overt toxic symptoms. This effect seems specific for lead and may result in a reduced clearance of particles from the lung (Bingham *et al.*, 1968). This would apply equally to bacteria as to any other particles inhaled.

C. Epidemiology of Lead with Other Diseases

There is considerable epidemiological evidence that morbidity and mortality are higher in areas with soft-water as compared with hard-water areas and the association is particularly evident when considering death from cardio-vascular disease (Kobayashi, 1957; Schroeder, 1960a, b, 1966; Morris *et al.*, 1961, 1962; Muss, 1962; Biorck *et al.*, 1965; Crawford and Crawford, 1967a) although some authors have failed to confirm this association (Lindemann and Assenzo, 1964). Mulcahahy (1964, 1966) reported no correlation but later recognized a trend when larger population samples were taken (Mulcahahy, 1968). There is no relationship between hard water and the development of atherosclerosis (Strong *et al.*, 1968).

Examining epidemiological and pathological data from patients dying from coronary artery disease in a soft-water district (Glasgow) and a hard-water district (London), Crawford and Crawford (1967) found that not only was a greater percentage of the Glasgow cases under fifty, but the pathological lesions were less marked than in the London cases, suggesting that there is a factor, or factors, altering the course of the disease in the soft-water area. The effect of lowered calcium in promoting lead uptake has stimulated a search for signs of increased lead absorption in persons dying from cardio-vascular disease. Crawford and Crawford (1969) found that rib lead content was higher in the Glasgow patients than in those from London. Morgan (1972), on the other hand, was unable to find any difference in renal lead concentration in patients with and without ischaemic heart disease.

Crawford *et al.* (1968) examined domestic water from a number of different boroughs and in all cases lead concentration was low. When the water had been allowed to remain overnight in the pipes then high values (over 0·3 ppm in some cases) were obtained in both hard- and soft-water districts (Crawford and Morris, 1967; Wilson, 1967). It is probable that factors other than lead are involved. For example, magnesium concentration in rib was slightly lower in the Glasgow cases and the concentrations of both calcium and magnesium were lower in the coronary arteries in cases under forty. Higher values were found in patients over this age, so that it may be that once the disease is established, these minerals are deposited in the lesions (Crawford and Crawford, 1967a). In addition, some workers have found that the correlation exists only between soft water and cardiovascular deaths in women (Boström and Webster, 1967; Biersteker, 1967) or between soft water and *sudden* death from ischaemic heart disease (Anderson *et al.*, 1969).

A survey of male civil servants in six soft-water and six hard-water towns has revealed that both diastolic and systolic blood pressure, heart rate (as shown by the R–R interval on the ECG) and plasma cholesterol are higher in the soft-water towns (Stitt *et al.*, 1973). Elwood and his colleagues (1971) by contrast found that P–R interval was longer in men from hard-water areas and that, in addition, they showed ventricular extrasystoles in a significantly higher proportion than men from soft-water districts.

In this complex situation where so many trace metals have been implicated (Maseroni, 1969) it is difficult to see what part lead plays, although it may be a substituent for calcium of magnesium in the heart muscle.

Lead has been implicated in the aetiology of cancer in an area of Devon where high concentrations of the metal have been found in the rocks, soil and foodstuffs (Allen-Price, 1960; Warren, 1963). Warren (1963, Warren *et al.*, 1967) has also suggested that it may be a causative factor in the production of multiple sclerosis. There is a relationship between soils having abnormally high concentrations of lead, zinc and copper and districts with an abnormally high incidence of multiple sclerosis. It has also been found that patients with multiple sclerosis have higher tooth lead concentrations than controls, indicating that their total body burden is greater (Campbell *et al.*, 1950).

Sterling (1964) has made some cautionary remarks concerning the epidemiology of diseases associated with lead, and has warned that correlation should not be taken to imply cause and effect. He has also commented that there are so many environmental factors to consider that it is difficult to select those which are truly correlated with disease from those which have a spurious correlation. These notes of caution should be observed; but, nevertheless, aetiological fashions, such as the viral aetiology of multiple sclerosis or dietary and stress factors in heart disease, should not blind scientists to the need to examine new correlations and devise means whereby they can be put to the test of experiment before rejecting them as spurious.

The multifactorial causation of disease is also a matter for consideration. In multiple sclerosis, for example, a slow virus theory does not necessarily exclude the possibility that other factors play a role in the aetiology. For example, interference by lead with the synthesis of myelin in early life may facilitate infection of nervous tissue by a virus, or alternatively, lead may encourage the infection by affecting immune mechanisms.

5 Diagnosis

I. SYMPTOMATOLOGY

There are no symptoms which are peculiar to lead poisoning and this can cause difficulties in diagnosis, particularly in children (Alexander and Delves, 1972). The lack of specificity of the symptoms of lead poisoning may result in the patient being admitted to a surgical ward and there is a real danger of coming to laparotomy (Mann, 1962). The diagnosis is often made with the knowledge of an immediate past exposure. The most common presenting symptoms in both inorganic and organic poisoning are shown in Table 42 which stresses the great difference between the

Table 42

A comparison of symptoms in inorganic and organic lead poisoning

INORGANIC		ORGANIC[c]
Adults[a]	Children[b]	
Abdominal pain	Drowsiness	Disturbances in sleep pattern
Constipation	Irritability	Nausea
Vomiting	Vomiting	Anorexia
Non-abdominal pain	Gastrointestinal symptoms	Vomiting
Asthenia	Ataxia	Vertigo and headache
Paraesthesiae	Stupor	Muscular weakness
Psychological symptoms	Fatigue	Weight loss
Diarrhoea		Tremor
		Diarrhoea
		Abdominal pain
		Hyperexcitability
		Mania

Symptoms are listed in their order of frequency as presenting symptoms
[a] Dagg *et al.* (1965)
[b] Sachs *et al.* (1970).
[c] Kehoe (1925), Cassells and Dodds (1946)

symptoms of the two different types. Psychological and neurological symptoms develop late in inorganic poisoning but are the earliest to appear in poisoning by organolead compounds and may include disturbances in personality and behaviour, whilst hallucinations are a common early manifestation. Inorganic lead poisoning may present with different symptoms in children as compared with adults. In children neurological symptoms are more common and this may be because children seem to expose themselves acutely to very high levels of lead (Chisholm and Harrison, 1956).

Progressive anorexia is an early sign in childhood lead poisoning. As the disease develops the child may become less playful, less alert and increasingly irritable. It may become clumsy or frankly ataxic. Vomiting may occur as may self-limiting episodes of convulsions. Constipation and colic are not usual although vague abdominal pain may be present. Encephalopathy is likely to develop if the disease is not diagnosed at an early stage and practitioners must have a high index of suspicion, especially when dealing with children under two years old in whom the disease can develop with particular rapidity (American Academy of Pediatrics, 1969). Symptoms not shown in Table 42 but which may also be present in the adult include headaches, arthralgia, dyspepsia and a metallic taste in the mouth.

The similarity between the symptomatology of lead poisoning and acute intermittent porphyria is well known (Dagg *et al.*, 1965) but biochemical investigations readily differentiate between the two conditions.

Pica, that is, the ingestion of materials not normally regarded as food is often associated with lead poisoning in children. It is not peculiar to this condition, however, and probably represents a normal phase in maturation. In more extreme forms, it may be associated with mental retardation when the phase may persist for an unusually long time and children who show this tendency are called scavengers. There is no evidence that children who contract lead poisoning through pica is have lower I.Q.s than the general population (Chisholm and Harrison, 1956) and their condition is incidental to their being in a lead-enriched environment.

II. SIGNS

In the classical case of lead poisoning in adults, it may be possible to see the blue line on the gums which is eponymously ascribed to Burton (1840) although it was described earlier by Tanquerel des Planches (1839). It is due to the presence of lead sulphide in the gingival margin and some degree of dental decay is essential for its production. Peripheral neuropathy, with or without wrist drop, may be a feature in serious cases. Encephalopathy may develop in a few instances in adults but is much more common in children. Clinical anaemia is an important finding in inorganic poisoning but not in organic poisoning (Beattie *et al.*, 1972c). Conversely, hypotension is common in the latter (Sanders, 1964).

Radiography of the long bones in children may show the presence of a lead line which is a line of increased radio-density in the metaphysis of the growing end of the bone (Fig. 49). It was formerly thought that this

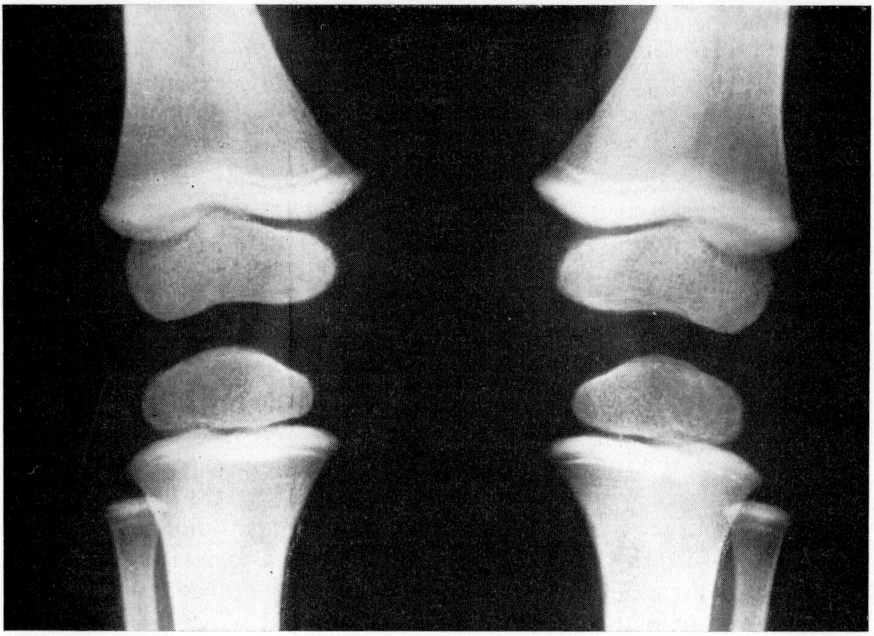

FIG. 49. Radiograph showing lead lines in the bones around the knee joint in a child with lead poisoning.

appearance was due to the lead deposited in this site (Vogt, 1930; Park *et al.*, 1933) but more recent work suggests that it is due to an increase in the calcium content of the bone brought about by the interference by lead with the normal process of resorption (Leone, 1968). All children presenting with an unexplained encephalopathy should have a radiographic examination for the presence of lead lines (Cooper, 1947). X-rays of the abdomen of children suspected of having ingested lead may also be helpful in showing radio-opaque material present in the gut (Fig. 50).

Greyish stippling of the retina has been described as an early sign of

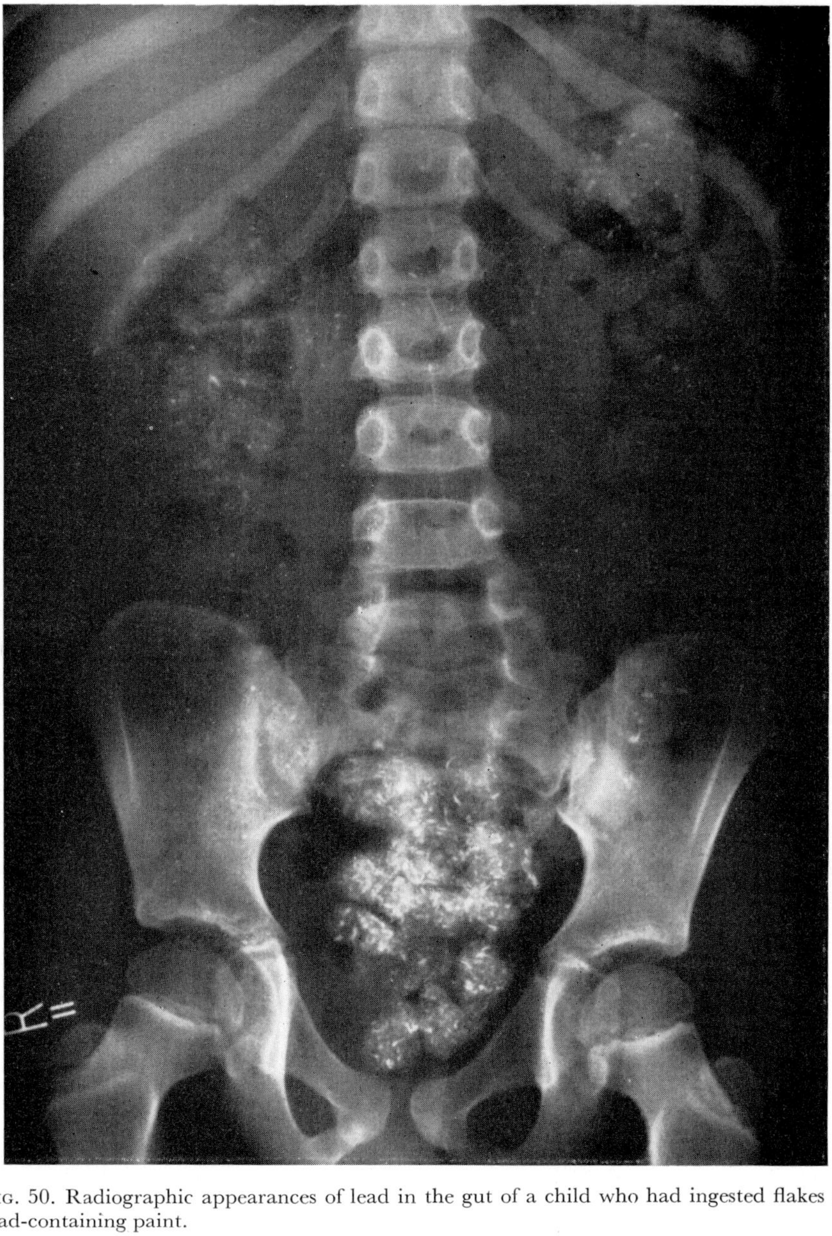

FIG. 50. Radiographic appearances of lead in the gut of a child who had ingested flakes of lead-containing paint.

lead poisoning (Sonkin, 1963). The stippling is found concentrated circumferentially around the optic disc. This observation has not been reported by other workers and was not noted in a series of patients with lead encephalopathy (Whitfield *et al.*, 1972), and its usefulness is thus open to doubt.

III. LABORATORY INVESTIGATIONS

Laboratory tests give an index either of lead absorption or of metabolic poisoning (Table 43). It is important to remember that in organic lead

Table 43

Tests of lead absorption and lead poisoning

Absorption	Poisoning
Blood lead	Urine ALA
Urine lead	Urine coproporphyrin
Faecal lead	Erythrocyte ALA-d
Hair lead	Erythrocyte protoporphyrin
Tooth lead	Haemoglobin
Lead mobilization	
Radiology	

poisoning there is no disturbance of porphyrin metabolism other than raised erythrocyte protoporphyrin in some instances. In addition, the blood lead may be normal or raised only slightly but urinary concentrations are higher than those seen in inorganic poisoning (Sanders, 1964).

There have been numerous studies made of the correlation between blood and urine lead concentrations as tests of absorption and urinary ALA, PBG and coproporphyrin excretion, and haemoglobin concentrations as indices of intoxication (Egli *et al.* 1957; Haeger-Aronsen, 1960; Stanković *et al.*, 1960; Kehoe, 1961a,b; King and Thompson, 1961; Stich, 1961; Buckup and Mappes, 1962; de Kretser and Waldron, 1963a; Albahary, 1964; Gattner and Schrantz, 1964; Meo *et al.*, 1964; Tsuchiya, 1964; Cramér and Selander, 1965; Balbo *et al.*, 1965; Williams, 1965; Djuric *et al.*, 1966; Selander *et al.*, 1966; Teisinger, 1966; Davis and Andelman, 1967; de Bruin and Holboom, 1967; Davis *et al.*, 1968; Gibson *et al.*, 1968; Rainsford, 1968; Singerman, 1964; Selander and Cramér, 1970; Urbanowicz, 1971; Waldron, 1971;

Zielhuis, 1971; Milic *et al.*, 1972; Prpic-Majic *et al.*, 1972; Soliman *et al.*, 1972). In general a good correlation is found between parameters of intoxication and absorption and in addition the laboratory tests correlate well with lead in air concentrations (Williams *et al.*, 1968, 1969; Azar *et al.*, 1972). The exceptions are that the haemoglobin level does not correlate well with other tests (Williams, 1966), nor does the punctate basophil count. The punctate basophil count enjoyed considerable popularity at one time particularly as a means of screening lead workers in industry through the work of Lane (1949) but has now fallen into disuse.

On the basis of published work and of experience, particularly in industry, guide-lines have been laid down for diagnosing lead poisoning (Lane *et al.*, 1968). Most workers, however, rely largely on the blood lead concentration to make the diagnosis and great weight has been given to Kehoe's statement that poisoning does not occur if the blood lead is less than 80 μg per cent (Kehoe, 1961a). There are objections, however, to making the diagnosis solely on the basis of the blood lead level (Danielson, 1969). Cases of poisoning have been reported with values less than this (Bénard *et al.*, 1950; Rossi, 1955; Jaulmes, 1962; Gibson *et al.*, 1968; Beritic, 1971; Beattie *et al.*, 1972a) and conversely, patients with extremely high blood leads may have minimal symptoms (Chamberlain and Massey, 1972; McRoberts, 1973). The occurrence of low (i.e. <80 μg) blood lead concentrations in cases of plumbism has been discussed by Kehoe (1972). He argues that this apparent anomaly is due to blood being sampled after exposure to lead has ceased and the concentration is falling so that it is below the threshold even though symptoms are still manifested by the patient. This argument is persuasive; but blood leads of less than 80 μg have been found in patients who were still exposed to the source (Beattie *et al.*, 1972a) and this raises doubts that it is the true explanation. It does not, of course, explain the finding of high blood levels without symptoms.

It has recently been suggested that the red cell/plasma partition of lead in the blood may be the determining factor in the development of toxic symptoms. In a small number of cases, symptoms were noted to occur when there was a shift in the partition towards an increase in the plasma concentration (McRoberts, 1973). The development of symptoms depends upon the concentration of lead in the soft tissues, and since this will be a function of the amount of diffusable lead in the plasma there seems much to commend this suggestion.

There is another objection to defining a blood lead concentration which arbitrarily delineates persons with lead poisoning from those without, apart from any sub-clinical considerations, and that is, that it does not seem possible to reproduce results from one laboratory to another. Inter-laboratory studies (Donovan *et al.*, 1971; Berlin *et al.*, 1972) have shown that there is an unacceptable large variation in the measurements made on the same sample by different centres. The results obtained are dependent to a large degree on the method used and some of the newer methods, such as polarography and atomic absorption, appear less reliable than the well established dithizone method (Keppler *et al.*, 1970; Hardy *et al.*, 1971). Other technical details, such as the failure to reduce the amount of ferric iron in the sample, may also add to the discrepancies (Millar *et al.*, 1970).

To define a threshold limit without taking such irregularities into account is clearly unsatisfactory. And neither does such a mandatory value allow for either the diurnal or seasonal variations which have been demonstrated (Vigliani, 1950; Suzutani and Taira, 1962; Hoschek, 1961).

The undue reliance on blood lead concentrations may have come into the literature because much of the original work on lead toxicology has been undertaken in an industrial setting. Blood lead estimations of an exposed group of industrial workers are of value in controlling absorption by indicating the degree of contamination in the working environment. In this respect, they are more reliable than urinary lead estimation because of the diurnal variations in urinary lead excretion (Molyneux, 1964) and because of the difficulties in obtaining a 24-hr urine specimen in industry. Neither of these tests gives any information about metabolic poisoning in individual cases and other investigations must be performed if this is needed.

More recently, hair lead levels have been used to identify persons with high exposure (Kopito *et al.*, 1967; Pueschel *et al.*, 1972) and it is said that when the concentration is above 100 μg/g or when there is more than a 2:1 ratio between the concentration of proximal and distal segments there is a need for further investigation. Care must be taken in interpreting the results of hair lead analyses because the concentration found is the sum of external and internal deposition and because the concentration varies along the length of the hair. Within these limitations, it has been found useful in screening populations of children and adults and in selecting those who need to be investigated more fully (Pueschel *et al.*, 1972; Speizer *et al.*, 1972), and Rüssel and Schöberl (1972) have investigated its use in veterinary work.

The lead content of deciduous teeth is greater in city children than in those living in suburban areas suggesting that it is a function of total exposure (Needleman *et al.*, 1972). It is not a practicable test to use for routine work, however.

As a screening procedure ALA-d activity in the erythrocytes has been shown to be a most sensitive method (see Ch. 4). ALA-d activity is depressed within hours of exposure to lead and there is a significant negative correlation between ALA-d activity and blood lead concentration. The method has been used for detecting exposure and poisoning in children and adults (Bonsignore *et al.*, 1965; Bonsignore, 1966; de Bruin, 1968; de Bruin and Jong-Heisterkamp, 1968; Nakao *et al.*, 1968; Hernberg and Nikkanen, 1970; Millar *et al.*, 1970; Weissberg *et al.*, 1971; Secchi *et al.*, 1972; Caccuri and Pecora, 1972; Hernberg *et al.*, 1969, 1970, 1972), but Haeger-Aronsen *et al.* (1971) consider it too sensitive a method for routine screening of lead workers.

In cases where there is some difficulty in arriving at a diagnosis or where some time has elapsed between the termination of exposure and investigation, the lead mobilization test has been utilized as an index of the total body burden (Reiders and Brieger, 1955; Teisinger and Srbová, 1959; Desoille *et al.*, 1957; Bastenier *et al.*, 1957; Zahorski and Myślak, 1957; Albahary *et al.*, 1958; Saita, 1959; Whitaker *et al.*, 1962; Teisinger, 1964, 1971; Williams *et al.*, 1966). The test consists of measuring 24-hr urinary excretion and then administering EDTA orally or intravenously and remeasuring the 24-hr urinary lead output. In both control subjects and those with lead exposure there is a rise in lead excretion following EDTA administration. Teisinger (1971) concludes that an excretion in excess of 2 mg in 24 hr after intravenous EDTA (or 1 mg in 24 hr when there has been no recent exposure) is evidence of a potentially hazardous body burden.

IV. NEUROLOGICAL TESTS

There have been a number of studies undertaken to investigate the possibility of using neurophysiological methods to detect early signs of lead poisoning. Lane and Lewy (1935) measured chronaxie in a large group of lead workers but the neural changes they found after exposure to lead appeared more slowly than basophilic stippling in the peripheral blood and they concluded that this measurement was of limited diagnostic aid. The most frequently measured parameter has been the maximal motor conduction velocity (MMCV) but the results obtained are conflicting. Some authors have found that the MMCV is decreased in a minority of cases (Bergamini and Sirbour, 1960; Sessa *et al.*, 1965) whilst others have reported no abnormal findings (Simpson *et al.*, 1964; Delwaide and Chantraine, 1965; Catton *et al.*, 1970). The difficulty in using this test is that the MMCV remains normal so long as some of the fibres with the fastest conduction time remain intact and it is thus not very sensitive. Measurement of the conduction velocity of the slower fibres, on the other hand, appears to be a much more precise method for detecting sub-clinical nerve damage (Seppäläinen and Hernberg, 1972) but this is not a method which would be applicable for routine examination and in general neurophysiological tests are of little value at the present time in diagnosing lead poisoning.

V. RECOMMENDATIONS FOR DIAGNOSIS

The greatest controversy in diagnosing lead poisoning revolves around the values which should be used to distinguish the pathological from the non-pathological case. In this book no such criteria will be laid down, principally because results from one laboratory are not directly comparable to those from another (Donovan *et al.*, 1971; Berlin *et al.*, 1972). A more profitable approach is for individual laboratories to establish their own reference values from a suitable reference population. The reference population should be defined accurately in terms of age, sex, place of residence, smoking habits and exposure to lead. Distribution of values can be established and the value of the case under investigation can be expressed in terms of standard deviations from the mean of the relevant reference population. Values varying by more than two standard deviations from the mean may be considered as diagnostically significant.

It is recommended that a diagnostic complex be used to establish the diagnosis in individual cases satisfying the following criteria.

(i) Signs or symptoms referable to lead poisoning must be present.
(ii) There must be a positive history of exposure to lead.
(iii) At least one parameter of both lead absorption and lead intoxication must vary significantly from the mean of the reference values.

6. Prophylaxis and Treatment

I. PROPHYLAXIS

A. Industrial Use

The elimination of the risks of lead poisoning would involve the total abolition of the use of lead commercially, a proposition which is scarcely practicable, especially in view of the great importance which the metal has to certain sectors of the economy. Its use in industry is subject to a number of legal checks and restraints. The responsibility for supervising lead works is split between the Factory Inspectorate and the Alkali and Clean Air Inspectorate, the latter being responsible solely for those processes which emit lead into the atmosphere. Medical and laboratory supervision of lead workers is also legislated for. In addition, the Factory Inspectorate issues a number of documents to assist those concerned with industrial hygiene and the care of the lead workers in controlling lead hazards together with recommendations for threshold limit values (TLV's) for airborne lead or safe limits of lead in blood and urine (Her Majesty's Factory Inspectorate, 1971a, b, c, 1972).

The TLV for the inorganic lead concentration in an industrial working atmosphere is accepted as 0·20 mg/m^3 in this country but in America the lower limit of 0·15 mg/m^3 is recommended (Table 44). These values are widely used throughout Western Europe but the countries of Eastern Europe set much lower maxima, reflecting their generally more cautious attitude towards the metal, based on their extensive toxicological experiments using animals exposed to various concentrations of lead for times corresponding to normal industrial working periods (Gusev, 1960; Bryce-Smith, 1972a).

The TLV is defined as the maximum concentration of atmospheric lead to which workers may be repeatedly exposed for a 40-hr working week with no adverse effects on their health.

There are a number of objections to this concept, the principal one being that no reference is given to particle size. The hazard to health of

Table 44

Maximum concentrations of lead compounds in the working environment by country

Country	Concentration, mg/m^3			
	Inorganic lead	Lead sulphide	Lead arsenate	Organic lead (As Pb)
Bulgaria	0·01	0·50		0·005
Czechoslovakia	0·05			
Finland	0·20		0·15	
Germany (Fed. Rep.)	0·20			
Great Britain	0·20		0·15	0·075
Hungary	0·02			0·005
Japan	0·15			0·075
Poland	0·05			
Rumania	0·10	0·50		0·01
U.A.R.	0·15			
U.S.A.	0·15		0·15	0·10 TEL[a] 0·15 TML[a]
U.S.S.R.	0·01			0·005
Yugoslavia	0·15			0·075

[a] As Pb-skin

From ILO/WHO Committee (1968) and H.M.F.I. (1972)

airborne lead is intimately related to its particle size which determines the ease of absorption through the lungs and clearly, some consideration ought to be given to this aspect of the problem. The TLV also makes the tacit assumption that exposure is constant throughout all the lead-working industries both collectively and individually and so ignores important factors such as variation in tidal volume and the number of hours actually worked in the leaded environment which may often be in excess of 40. There is also a danger that the TLV may be looked upon as a permissive recommendation such that all concentrations up to the TLV are tolerated and it becomes a minimum safety level.

It is important to note that the industrial TLV applies only to adult males. Employment of women in lead industries is discouraged and employment of pregnant women and persons under eighteen years of age is not allowed by the Factory Inspectorate. The application of industrial TLV's to whole populations when assessing health hazards from airborne lead is thus inadmissable.

The biochemical guidelines of the Factory Inspectorate are also open to criticism, particularly the rigid adherence to absolute values for defining criteria of safety or hazard. Nevertheless, the control of lead hazards in industry has significantly reduced morbidity and mortality although incidents of excessive pollution are still reported (Ireland, 1972). Growing interest in lead pollution amongst the public at large has resulted in a number of incidents gaining notoriety in the press and in one case, the establishment of a Committee of Enquiry (Windeyer Committee, 1972). Experience also reveals that some compounds constitute more of a hazard than was at one time supposed. The most recent example is lead stearate which is now recognized as a much more toxic substance than was hitherto thought (Lloyd-Davies, 1972). These reports emphasize the need for stringent control of lead working processes and for reviewing existing standards in the light of current research.

B. Domestic Prophylaxis

1. *Food and Drink*

The lead content of food and drink is to some extent regulated by legislation (Table 45). There is in general, however, inadequate control so

Table 45

Statutory requirements or recommendations regarding the maximum lead content of various items in Great Britain

Food	2 ppm[a]
	5 ppm for tinned foods[a]
	0·5 ppm for tinned baby foods[b]
Water	0·1 ppm
Paint	5000 ppm in dry film on childrens' toys[c]
	1·5% in dry film in lead free or low in lead paints
Tinning on cooking utensils	2000 ppm[d]
Glazes	7 ppm extractable lead

[a] Lead in Food Regulations (1961): Statutory Instrument 1931
[b] Lead in Food Amendment Regulations (1972): Statutory Instrument 1843
[c] Toys (Safety) Regulations (1967): Statutory Instrument 1157
[d] Cooking Utensils (Safety) Regulations (1972): Statutory Instrument 1957

that there are opportunities for considerable contamination of foodstuffs and other domestic items to which the public unwittingly expose themselves, sometimes with serious results. Glazed earthenware is notorious as a source of lead in food and drink; reports of cases of lead poisoning, including some fatalities, following the use of earthenware vessels to prepare home-made wine or simply for storing food and drink are not uncommon (Whitehead and Prior, 1960; Beritić and Stahuljak, 1961; Harris and Elsea, 1967; Klein *et al.*, 1970, Clark, 1972; Williams, 1972). In the report of Klein and his colleagues, half the earthenware items tested yielded up more than 7 ppm of lead, and glazes on pottery and metal casseroles subjected to analysis by Bugler and Doyle (1972, 1973) also contained excessive amounts of lead in some instances.

Adulteration of other items of domestic use sometimes results in cases of poisoning from unusual sources including eye cosmetics (Warley *et al.*, 1968; Alexander and Delves, 1972), chilli powder (Power *et al.*, 1969) and an ointment for use on bunions (Srivastava and Umadi, 1968). Opium smoking may sometimes be additionally hazardous to the addict when the drug is prepared in vessels rich in lead (Chia *et al.*, 1973).

Lead in individual foods is subject to great variation as shown in the Appendix. The use of organic insecticides in place of lead arsenate is an important factor in minimizing the lead content of agricultural and horticultural crops. Some technological processes can increase the lead content of food and drink but contamination is less than it was mainly because of the substitution of other metals for lead in the food industry (Oser, 1970). Canning sometimes increases the lead content of food as was the case in some brands of baby food (Ministry of Agriculture, 1972); but leaching from soldered can seams is small (Bergner and Miethke, 1964) and few of a large number of samples of canned beef tested, some after many years in tins, were found to exceed the statutory 5 ppm (Government Chemist, 1968).

The regulations governing lead in food show some curious anomalies (Table 45). For example, what can be the justification for allowing tinned foods to contain more lead than fresh foods? Again, if 0·5 ppm is the limit for tinned baby foods, how is it possible to reconcile this with the higher limits permitted in other foods which babies are liable to eat?

The World Health Organization recommendation for the maximum lead content of drinking water is 0·1 ppm with the rider that the lead content must not exceed 0·3 ppm after 16-hr contact with the pipes (World Health Organization, 1971). Water distributed in Great Britain still complies with the earlier World Health Organization European limit of 0·05 ppm (World Health Organization, 1970; Egan, 1972). This value is often exceeded, however, because of the use of lead pipes in domestic water systems and may give rise to cases of poisoning (Bacon *et al.*, 1967; Parry, 1967; Beattie *et al.*, 1972a). In soft-water areas the use of lead pipes is particularly dangerous because the acidity of the water increases its facility for dissolving the metal and the low concentration of calcium impairs the formation of a calcium carbonate layer, which in hard-water districts, lines the pipes and impedes solution of the lead. Reed and Tolley (1967a,b) showed that a large number of localities in Britain had waters which were of a low enough pH to dissolve lead and incapable of forming calcium carbonate. They suggested that no domestic water should be allowed to have a calcium carbonate content below 100 mg/litre where lead pipes were in use in order that the plumbosolvent properties of the water should be kept to a minimum (Reed and Tolley, 1967c).

Wilson (1965, 1967) has mentioned other factors which increase the lead content of drinking water including the use of lead storage tanks, the joining of copper and lead pipes or earthing electric wires to lead pipes, both of which increase the solution of lead through electrolysis. He has also noted that differences in lead content of drinking water may vary from house to house within one region as a function of the total length of lead piping which the water traverses. Moore (1973) has shown how critical the factors of pH and temperature are in determining the plumbosolvency of water. He has also drawn attention to the fact that old lead pipes are often deeply fissured so that they present a much greater surface area than new pipes of the same nominal diameter. In some areas polyphosphates are added to drinking water to prevent the precipitation of metals such as iron and manganese, but under some conditions they have been shown to increase plumbosolvency (Baydens, 1957). Plastic pipes are not entirely free from hazard because lead stearate is becoming increasingly used as a filler. Water left undisturbed for several hours in new polyvinyl chloride pipes was found to contain high concentrations of lead (300–1,000 μg/litre after 6 hr) and did not fall to acceptable levels until the pipes had been used for several days. Water from old plastic pipes contains lead in low concentrations (Packham, 1971).

The World Health Organization has recommended that the maximum daily intake of lead from food and drink should not be in excess of 5 μg/kg/day (World Health Organization, 1971). The intake of lead from food varies very widely (Thompson, 1971) and it is easy to see that this figure might readily be approached by adults particularly in areas where soft drinking water is taken from leaden pipes. For a 70 kg man the intake should not be greater than 350 μg. The Ministry of Agriculture Report (1972) estimates that the average intake from food and beverages is 220 μg; assuming that 2·5 litres of water is drunk in addition with a lead concentration of 50 μg/litre, then this gives another 125 μg, and a total of 345 μg. If the new World Health Organization limit on water of 100 μg/litre should be adopted, then the daily permissible limit could easily be surpassed. Amphlett-Williams (1972) has pointed out that the adoption of the new World Health Organization limit of 100 μg/litre could have an even more undesirable effect on the total lead exposure of young children.

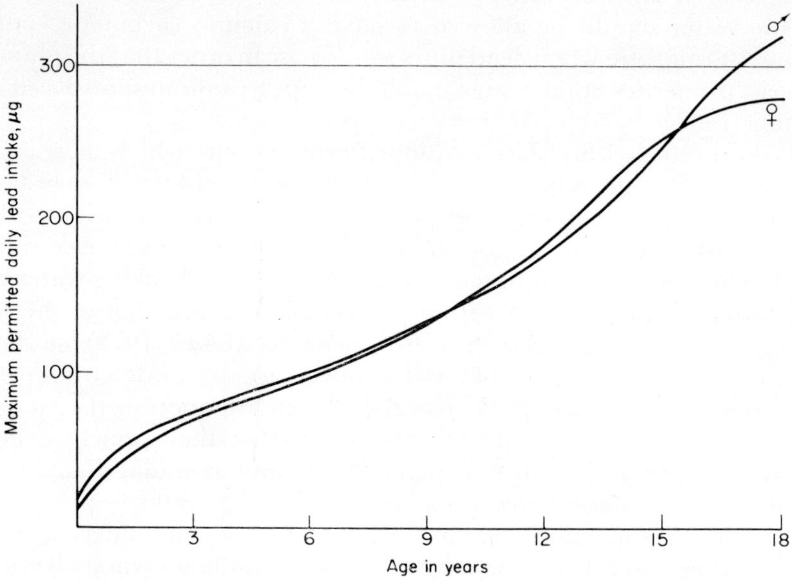

Fig. 51. Graph showing maximum permitted daily intake of lead for children up to the age of eighteen. Points on the graph are calculated from 50th percentile of standard growth and development charts and WHO recommendation of 5 μg Pb/kg/day. Horizontal line shows the upper limit of 300 μg/day recommended by King (1971).

King (1971) has proposed that the maximum daily intake in children which will not result in an excessive body burden is 300 μg. This figure is at odds with the World Health Organization recommendation which it exceeds greatly until both boys and girls are post-pubertal (Fig. 51). This is not to say that King's recommendation is therefore dangerous, but because blanket maxima tend to become regarded as minimum safety requirements, it seems safer to link all such proposals to body weight.

To safeguard the public, it seems advisable to ban entirely the use of lead in glazes on cooking ware and crockery, and to establish a statutory limit of 50 μg lead/litre for drinking water at the tap. In addition, it would be desirable to ban polyphosphate additives and to add calcium to soft water as suggested by Reed and Tolley and, where necessary, remove organic acids whilst lead is a constituent of domestic water systems. A more fundamental approach would be for improvement grants to be made available to permit people to replace lead drinking pipes in their homes. It might be in the public interest to show the lead content on packaged foods so that the public could choose those which were low in lead if they so desired.

2. *Lead in Air*

Although some countries have proposed maxima for ambient lead concentrations (Table 46) there is no legislation governing the concentration of lead in the atmosphere in this country and there is much debate, both in Britain and America, as to what constitutes a potential threat. The United States Environmental Protection Agency (1972) considers that

Table 46

Recommended ambient air quality standards for inorganic lead

Country	Concentration mg Pb/m^3	Averaging time
Canada		
Ontario	0·02	30 minutes
Czechoslovakia	0·0007	24 hours
East Germany	0·0007	24 hours
West Germany[a]	0·001–0·003	
U.S.A.[b]	0·002	3 months
Montana	0·005	30 days
Pennsylvania	0·005	30 days
U.S.S.R.	0·0007	24 hours
	0·0017[c]	24 hours

[a] Proposed by VDI–Kommission Reinhaltung der Luft, Düsseldorf
[b] Proposed by Environmental Protection Agency
[c] Standard for PbS (as Pb)

Based in part on Stern (1968).

air lead levels greater than 2 $\mu g/m^3$ averaged over a period of 3 months or more are associated with sufficient risk of adverse physiological effects that they constitute a danger to public health. Goldsmith (1969) has proposed that levels of 2 $\mu g/m^3$ are the most which are compatible with safety but Goldwater (1972) has raised this to 4 $\mu g/m^3$ and Kehoe (1969)

Table 47

Permitted levels of lead in petrol

Country	Present limit g/l	Proposed future limits	Lead-free petrol by
Australia	0·84		
Austria	0·4		
Belgium	0·84		
Denmark	0·85		
France	0·64		
Germany (Fed. Rep.)	0·4	0·15 from 1976	
Italy	0·635		
Japan	0·29	Zero by 1974	1974
The Netherlands	0·84		
Norway	0·7		
Sweden	0·4	0·15 from 1976	1977
Switzerland	0·57 premium 0·54 regular		
South Africa	0·84		
Great Britain	0·84	0·45 from 1976	
U.S.A.—Federal	1·1	0·53 from 1974 0·45 from 1975 0·40 from 1976 0·33 from 1977	
—New York	0·27	0·13 from 1973 Zero from 1974	
U.S.S.R.	Zero in main cities		

Based on Blackmore (1972) and Barry and Harrison (1972)

considers that below 10 μg/m^3 there is no progressive accumulation of lead in the body. The contrast between Western and Eastern standards is interesting here, for the Russians set a limit of 0·7 μg/m^3 based on their toxicological studies (Rjazanov, 1965). Since the mean atmospheric lead concentration in many European and American cities is greater than 2 μg/m^3 (Table 4) it is clearly a matter of some urgency that the difference of opinion which is currently displayed by western authorities should be resolved.

The removal of lead from petrol would undoubtedly have an effect in lowering ambient lead levels in cities and many countries have now acted to reduce maximum levels of lead in petrol and in some cases, introduced legislation to provide for lead-free petrol (Table 47). It is important to realize, however, that the concentration of lead in petrol is not *per se* of any significance but rather it is the total amount of lead alkyl put into petrol each year, and it is this which should be controlled if a serious effort is to be made to reduce lead emission from motor-cars. As an interim measure, the use of alumina filters on car exhausts which are said to remove up to 60 or 70 per cent of lead from the exhaust gases (Barry and Harrison, 1972) might be considered. These have the added advantage that it might be possible to remove the lead from them. Filters presently under discussion would not, however, remove organolead from exhaust gases in any appreciable amounts.

3. *Paint*

Lead in paint comes from two sources, from compounds used as pigments and, in the case of oil paints, from the use of lead naphthenate as a drier. There is a statutory limit of 5,000 ppm in the dry film of paint used on children's toys but no legislation exists otherwise to govern the use of lead in paint. Paint technology has advanced to the point that there are now many alternative compounds which can replace lead, and many lead-free or low-in-lead paints are available. To conform with the British Standards Specification, paints described as lead-free or low-in-lead should contain a maximum of 1·5 per cent of lead in the dry film. These paints are considered by the B.S.I. as suitable for use on surfaces likely to be chewed by children.

A survey in Birmingham by the city analyst showed that many paints on sale had a high lead content (Coombes, 1972). Lead primers contained from 3·0 to 62·7 per cent, although most gave warnings about use on surfaces which might be chewed by children. All the lead-free primers contained less than one per cent of lead, range nil to 0·96 per cent, and the content in coloured paints ranged from nil to 7·3 per cent. In many cases, there was no warning notice on the can that the paint contained lead.

It is unfortunately common-place that in an attempt to minimize the dangers of leaded paints to children, parents cover the leaded surface with lead-free paints, assuming that this is an adequate safeguard. Children with pica, however, often chew painted surfaces down to the wood and so ingest all the layers of paint which cover it (Fig. 52). To be safe it is necessary to strip all surfaces to the bare wood and use only primers, undercoats and topcoats which are lead free.

To provide ideal protection, paints should contain no lead at all. The greatest technological difficulty is in providing an alternative to lead naphthenate as a drier since there are now sufficient non-toxic pigments to replace lead compounds. The level of 1·5 per cent in the B.S.S. for low-in-lead paints seems high. In the New York child screening programme, if a child is shown to have a blood lead concentration in excess

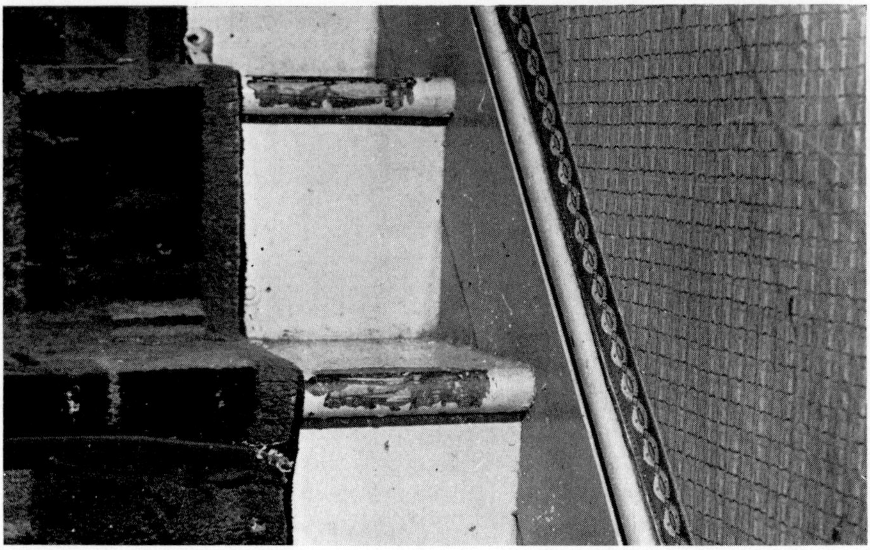

FIG. 52. The effects of pica on stairs. The paint contained 0·9 per cent lead.

of 60 μg/100 ml the house is visited and samples of paint analysed. Should the paint contain more than one per cent of lead, the owner is required to replace it within five days (Guinee, 1972). Since 1st January, 1973 the Food and Drug Administration of America has banned the use of paints containing more than 0·5 per cent of lead by weight on residential surfaces accessible to children, and Great Britain would be wise to benefit from the American experience and introduce similar measures.

4. *Individual Susceptibility*

Prophylactic measures should take some account of individual susceptibility. This can be defined as an undue sensitivity on the part of an individual to the toxic effects of lead. It may result either from personal idiosyncrasy or because concomitant dietary deficiencies or diseases act to enhance the toxic effects. Writers in the last century and the early part of the present century made much of the former condition. It is undoubtedly a real phenomenon and there is some slight evidence to support the view that it may be genetically determined. Legge and Goadby (1912) and Oliver (1914), in their classic works, recorded instances in which more than one member of the family appeared unduly susceptible and Lane and Lewy (1935) described three brothers as having this trait. One of the three had suffered from mild lead poisoning and the other two rapidly produced high stippled cell counts on exposure to lead. After removal from lead work the stippled cell counts quickly fell to normal. The youngest brother was again exposed to lead whereupon his stippled cell count once more became markedly elevated and he was removed from further exposure.

Concomitant factors which have been implicated at one time or another include age, season, dietary intake of calcium, phosphate, iron, protein, vitamins C and D, nicotinic acid, alcohol and other metals and co-existing disease (Goyer and Mahaffey, 1972). Impaired renal excretion may also be important (Bryce-Smith, 1972a).

The effects of age, season and the intake of calcium, phosphate and vitamin D have all been considered elsewhere. Suffice it to say that children seem more prone to lead poisoning than adults and that most cases in childhood occur in the summer. In view of the frequent association of iron deficiency in children with plumbism, it is interesting to note that iron-deficient rats have been found to have greater body burdens of lead than those with an adequate iron intake (Six and Goyer, 1972). Diets low in cystine, methionine and casein appear to enhance the toxic effects of lead (Baernstein and Grand, 1942; Gontzea *et al.*, 1964a). The position of the relation between ascorbic acid and lead toxicity is presently uncertain. Some authorities have reported that there is no effect one upon the other (Dannenberg *et al.*, 1940; Evans *et al.*, 1943), whereas others consider that lead increases vitamin C requirements in both humans and animals exposed to it (Gontzea *et al.*, 1963, 1964b).

Alcoholics are apparently more susceptible to the effects of lead than others (Cramér, 1966) and it is in their interests not to work in a lead industry. Persons with thalassaemia and G-6-PD deficiency should also not be accepted as lead workers (Stokinger and Mountain, 1967; Albahary, 1972). Patients with kidney disease face an increased risk of toxic effects from ingested lead and should be protected from it as far as it is possible (Tange *et al.*, 1965).

5. *The Place of Milk in Prophylaxis*

Milk has been used as a prophylactic measure in lead industries for many years and is still advocated by Hunter (1969). The origins of the practice are undiscernable and it was probably an empirical observation, most likely owing its effectiveness to correcting dietary imbalance of calcium and phosphate. Since calcium concentration in the gut is a factor of importance with respect to lead absorption, it is reasonable to suppose that milk might decrease the amount of lead taken up. Wittgens and Niederstadt (1954, 1955) published the results of experiments with rats which indicated that the addition of milk to the diets of these animals actually increased the toxic effects of lead. These results have gained wide credence although similar experiments conducted by Ardelean *et al.* (1955) produced exactly opposite findings.

The provision of milk for children, who are the group most at risk of developing lead poisoning, is of more importance nowadays than its use in industry if only because the children who have the greatest exposure come from the lowest social groups and are most likely to have dietary deficiencies. Children with poor calcium intake are likely to absorb more lead from the gut than if dietary calcium were adequate. It would be in the interest of public health to ensure adequate calcium intake by encouraging increased milk consumption or by the use of calcium supplements.

II. TREATMENT

The use of chelating agents is now the treatment of choice in lead poisoning. The heavy metals can, for the most part, be divided into two classes, those which preferentially bind to either O or N or S or P in chelating agents and it is this which dictates the drug to be used in therapy. Lead is the exception in that it will bind to all four groups and any of the available chelating agents is effective.

Three drugs are in use, BAL, calcium—EDTA and D-penicillamine. Lead forms a complex with each and their chemical configurations are depicted in Figs. 53–55. The Pb—EDTA and Pb—penicillamine complexes are excreted solely in the urine whereas the Pb—BAL complexes are excreted in both the urine and the faeces depending whether it is the polar or non-polar form which is produced.

A. BAL (Dimercaprol, 2:3 dimercapto-1-propanol)

BAL is not properly a chelating agent but owes its effectiveness to its —SH groups for which lead has a great affinity. The Pb—BAL complex is a ring structure in which the metallic ions are bound in a relatively stable form.

The drug was originally produced as an antidote for the war gas lewisite, an arsenical vesicant, and was known as British-Anti-Lewisite (Peters *et al.*, 1945). It was found to be effective in experimental lead poisoning in animals (Braun *et al.*, 1946; Chiodi and Sammartino, 1947; Weatherall, 1948) but initial reports of its effectiveness in humans were not encouraging (Ryder *et al.*, 1947; Telfer, 1947). Later its place in the management of the disease was established (Foreman, 1955; Giannattasio, 1956; Brieger, 1960); but it has been largely superseded by EDTA

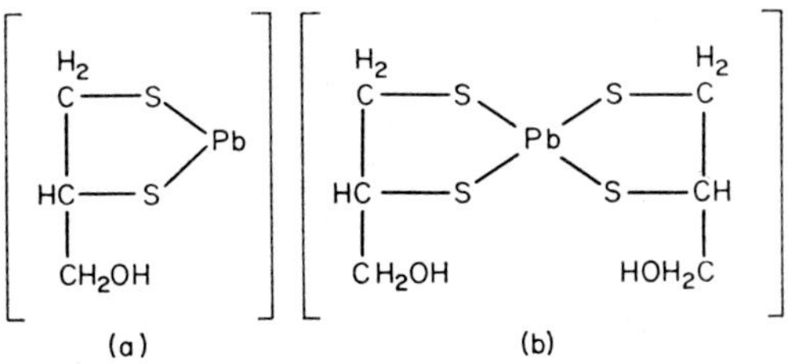

FIG. 53. Formula of Pb—BAL complexes, (a) non-polar, (b) polar forms.

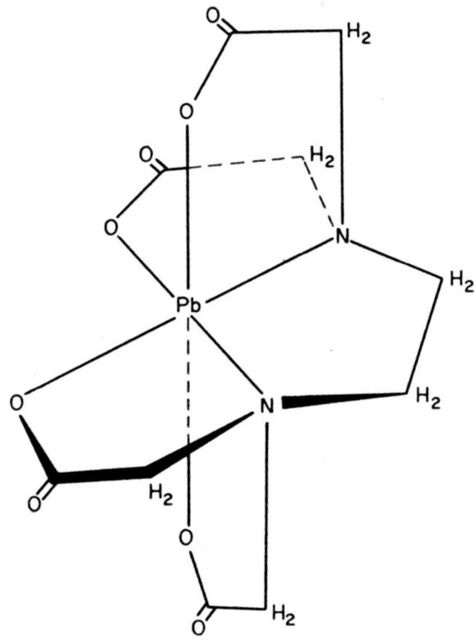

FIG. 54. Formula of Pb—EDTA complex.

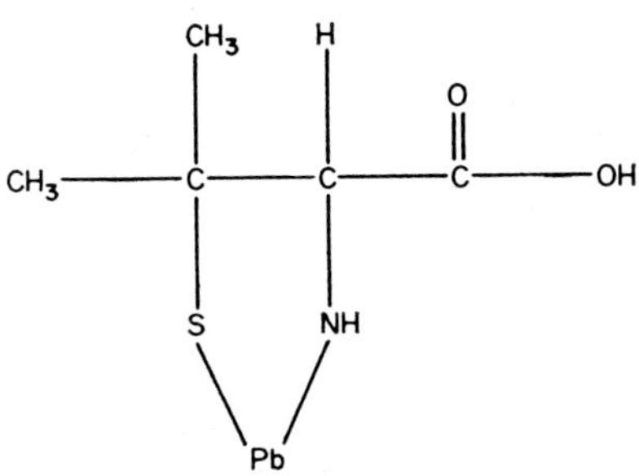

FIG. 55. Formula of Pb—penicillamine complex.

and penicillamine, although some authorities still consider it has a place either singly or in combination with EDTA (Chisholm, 1968).

Hepatic but not renal damage is a contraindication to the use of BAL and the drug can only be given by deep intramuscular injection. Toxic side-effects include lacrimation, blepharospasm, paraesthesiae, nausea, tachycardia and hypertension (Stocken and Thompson, 1949).

The recommended dosage schedule is outlined in Table 48.

Table 48

Dosage schedules for treatment of lead poisoning

Drug	Dose	Route	Contraindications
BAL	18 mg/kg/24 hr for 2 days 12 mg/kg/24 hr for 1 day 6 mg/kg/24 hr for 7 days	Deep i.m.	Hepatic disease
Ca-EDTA	50 mg/kg/24 hr for 5 days Allow 2 days before starting a second course	I.V. or I.M.	Kidney disease
D-penicillamine	0·9–1·5 g/24 hr	Oral	Kidney disease

B. EDTA (Ethylenediamine Tetra-acetic Acid)

EDTA was introduced as a treatment for lead poisoning in both adults and children in 1952 (Belknap, 1952; Bessman *et al.*, 1952) and has since become widely accepted as the drug of first choice. Although it may be given orally, the best results are obtained when it is administered parenterally.

Adequate urine flow must be established before the drug is given and renal damage is a contraindication to its use.

Side effects are common and include lacrimation, nasal congestion, sneezing, muscular pains and hypotension. Kidney damage, including tubular necrosis is a more serious hazard but is fortunately not common. Long-term oral dosage has been accompanied by a number of poorly defined effects including chelosis, rashes and fevers (Dudley *et al.*, 1955; Foreman, 1963).

The dosage schedule is set out in Table 48. The maximal safe dose is usually considered to be 75 mg/kg/24 hr, although even this dose is not without some risk (Foreman *et al.*, 1956) and some authorities recommend that 50 mg/kg/24 hr should not be exceeded (Chisholm, 1970). It is imperative that the calcium salt is given to avoid the possibility of hypocalcaemia and tetany.

C. D-penicillamine ($\beta\beta$-dimethylcysteine)

Penicillamine is a degradation product of penicillin and was first used therapeutically as a copper chelator in Wilson's disease (Walshe, 1956). Its effectiveness in increasing urinary copper excretion suggested that it might be useful also in lead poisoning and it was introduced quickly into the therapeutic arsenal (Boulding and Baker, 1957; Harris, 1958).

Side effects include leucopaenia, neutropaenia, defects in coagulation, rashes, altered collagen metabolism and fever at high doses. The drug also combines with pyridoxine and pyridoxine deficiency may occur. It is also nephrotoxic. At doses of 40 mg/kg/day of the free base, or 50 mg/kg/day of the hydrochloride, side effects are minimal, and this dose is recommended if long-term administration is required (Gibbs and Walshe, 1966).

Chronic renal damage is a contraindication to its use and, although cross-sensitization has not been convincingly demonstrated, care should be taken when giving the drug to patients known to have an allergy to penicillin.

The drug is given orally, preferably on an empty stomach. The dosage schedule is set out in Table 48.

D. General Comments on Treatment

To be effective, the treatment of lead poisoning requires the administration of a significant molar excess of chelating agent over lead. This is of prime importance when treating children with encephalopathy and the highest dose which is consistent with safety should be given. If inadequate doses are given, there is evidence that the effect is merely to redistribute the metal in the body and its toxic effects may be increased (Chisholm, 1968).

Toxic symptoms may also be exacerbated if chelating agents are given to children with paint chips in the gastro-intestinal tract since the lead in the gut may be solubilized.

When dealing with patients suspected of having lead poisoning, and especially children with encephalopathy, it is best to err on the side of prompt treatment rather than wait for the results of confirmatory laboratory tests.

During treatment, patients should be monitored by daily total urinary lead excretion and blood lead concentrations. Serum calcium, phosphorus and urea should also be checked regularly.

Summary and Conclusions

1. There can be no doubt that human industry has increased the mobilization of lead into the environment and that this contamination has increased since the Industrial Revolution. The use of lead alkyls in petrol has added considerably to the burden of lead in the environment and constitutes the major source of lead in the atmosphere of cities.

2. Mortality and morbidity from classical lead poisoning have decreased during this century largely due to improve industrial hygiene and better care of the lead worker. Despite this, cases of industrial poisoning still occur and there are lapses in safety standards from time to time in lead industries which constitute a threat to the health both of those employed and of the public at large.

3. The danger to children from leaded paint is sufficiently serious to consider barring absolutely the use of lead in paint and because of the danger to the public at large, it seems desirable to restrict the use of lead in glazes.

4. Lead in domestic water may cause frank poisoning on occasion, especially in soft water districts and it seems reasonable that all domestic water should be treated in such a way as to reduce its plumbosolvency to a minimum and ensure that it is able to form a protective calcium carbonate coat on lead piping. It might also be advisable to make the World Health Organization European standard of 0·05 ppm of lead in drinking water a statutory limit.

There is a strong case for barring the installation of lead pipes for drinking water and for awarding public grants for the removal of existing pipes and water cisterns. The use of lead solders to seal and join copper pipes can cause the release of lead through galvanic action and should be prohibited.

5. Although the maximum lead content of food is fixed by law, there is a very wide variation in the lead concentration of different foods and it would be in the public interest to require manufacturers to show the maximum lead content on the package so that foods low in lead could be bought preferentially if desired.

The present legal maximum of 2 ppm for untinned foodstuffs should be revised downwards and the anomalies in the regulations clarified, preferably by adopting for all foods the lowest limit presently in force (i.e. 0·5 ppm).

6. Present levels of lead in the environment constitute a well recognized health hazard to children, particularly those living in sub-standard urban housing. Chewing lead paint is a frequent cause of the cases of overt clinical poisoning which bring children to hospital. Up to 25 per cent of children screened in some poorer areas of American cities are authoritatively reported to have potentially dangerous amounts of lead in their blood, and up to 5 per cent show symptoms of lead poisoning. Some more limited studies suggest that a comparable problem exists in the United Kingdom. Tap water contaminated by lead is now recognized as a special problem in some soft-water areas of Britain. The early symptoms of lead poisoning are protean and non-specific so that they may be confused easily with those of other disorders. Thus the true incidence of lead poisoning in a particular locality may not be apparent unless medical workers have been alerted and trained to recognize the disease. Most adults in cities have blood lead levels below those which are at present known to be associated with a risk of clinical lead poisoning. However, the safety margin is less than for any other recognized chemical pollutant and raises the possibility, as yet unproven, that adverse effects on behaviour, mentation and chronic disease states may be occurring among the general population. A considerable corpus of data derived from experimental studies on animals shows that both morbidity and mortality can be increased by the administration of lead in doses insufficient to cause clinical symptoms of lead poisoning. In addition, biochemical and morphological changes have been observed in human subjects exposed to lead but without overt plumbism and there is some evidence that behavioural changes may also be brought about by low concentrations of lead.

There is sufficient evidence to justify the conclusion that city dwellers are exposed to higher levels of ambient lead than those living in rural areas but the concentration of lead in the atmosphere which constitutes a long-term threat to health is yet to be established, but levels reported for the vicinity of main roads in the United Kingdom are often higher than the maximum levels officially considered safe by public health authorities in America and Russia.

7. There is no justification in assuming that individuals are in a state of lead balance in view of the unequivocal evidence that the total body burden of lead rises with age due mainly to increasing skeletal deposition. Increased dissemination of lead into the environment is certain to add

to the body burden by increasing exposure through the air and the diet. There is ample evidence that lead has metabolic effects at levels which are insufficient to produce clinical symptoms and so it is expedient to reduce lead exposure to a minimum and to re-assess currently accepted limits of lead concentrations in the body compartments.

There is an urgent need to establish whether present-day environmental levels of lead are producing harmful physiological or psychological effects particularly in children, who are most at risk. It would also be prudent to initiate studies among special groups from the adult population, including those having certain categories of chronic disease and perhaps those showing behavioural abnormalities consistent with the known long-term effects of lead on higher nervous function.

Appendix

LEAD IN FOOD AND DRINK

Item	Country of Origin[a]	Lead Content ppm	Authors
Cereals and Grains			
Barley heads		0·5–2·0	Warren and Delavault (1962)
Corn	U.S.A.	0	Kehoe *et al.* (1933c)
Corn grain	U.S.A.	0·03–0·33	Kehoe *et al.* (1940b)
Maize seedling	Brit.Columbia	0·3–18·0	Warren and Delavault (1962)
Oat heads	Brit. Columbia	0·3–2·0	Warren and Delavault (1962)
Oat ears		0·5–6·0	Warren and Delavault (1962)
Rice	U.S.A.	0	Kehoe *et al.* (1933c)
Rice	India	0	Bagchi *et al.* (1940)
Rice		0·4	Monier-Williams (1938)
Rye heads		0·3–7·0	Warren and Delavault (1962)
Wheat grain	U.S.A.	0·27–0·4	Kehoe *et al.* (1940b)
Wheat head		1·0—2·0	Warren and Delavault (1962)
Cereals		0·27	Tolan and Elton (1972)
Flour, three types		<0·01–0·22	Min. of Agriculture (1972)
Flour		2·4	Monier-Williams (1938)
Bread	U.S.A.	0·0–0·16	Kehoe *et al.* (1933c)
Bread, white		<0·01–0·22	Min. of Agriculture (1972)
Bread, non-white		<0·01–0·33	Min. of Agriculture (1972)
Bread, white	U.S.A.	0·02–0·16	Kehoe *et al.* (1940b)
Bread, white		0·2	Monier-Williams (1938)
Bread, white	India	0·2	Bagchi *et al.* (1940)
Vegetables			
Asparagus	U.S.A.	0·60	Kehoe *et al.* (1933c)
Beans, string, frozen	U.S.A.	0·01	Schroeder and Balassa (1961)

[a] Great Britain unless otherwise stated.

Item	Country of Origin	Lead Content ppm	Authors
Vegetables (*contd.*)			
Beans, green, frozen		0·01–0·03	Min. of Agriculture (1972)
Beans, broad, frozen		0·02–0·08	Min. of Agriculture (1972)
Beans, string, canned	U.S.A.	0·03	Schroeder and Balassa (1961)
Beans	U.S.A.	0·15–0·26	Kehoe *et al.* (1940b)
Beans, kidney, dried	U.S.A.	0·16	Schroeder and Balassa (1961)
Beans, runner		0·3	Monier-Williams (1938)
Beet	U.S.A.	0	Kehoe *et al.* (1933c)
Beet	India	0·21	Bagchi *et al.* (1940)
Beet, root	Brit. Columbia	1·0–6·0	Warren and Delavault (1962)
Beet, root		1·0–6·0	Warren and Delavault (1962)
Beet, root	U.S.A.	3·0–4·0	Kehoe *et al.* (1940b)
Broccoli, frozen	U.S.A.	0·03	Schroeder and Balassa (1961)
Broccoli, frozen		0·03–0·08	Min. of Agriculture (1972)
Brussels sprouts	U.S.A.	0	Kehoe *et al.* (1933c)
Brussels sprouts		<0·01–0·24	Min. of Agriculture (1972)
Brussels sprouts, frozen		0·03–0·08	Min. of Agriculture (1972)
Cabbage, white	U.S.A.	0	Schroeder and Balassa (1961)
Cabbage, red	U.S.A.	0	Schroeder and Balassa (1961)
Cabbage		<0·01–0·51	Min. of Agriculture (1972)
Cabbage	U.S.A.	0·10–0·24	Kehoe *et al.* (1933c)
Cabbage	U.S.A.	0·10–0·24	Kehoe *et al.* (1940b)
Carrots		<0·01–0·04	Min. of Agriculture (1972)
Carrots	India	0·24–0·29	Bagchi *et al.* (1940)
Carrots		2·0	Warren and Delavault (1962)
Carrots	U.S.A.	2·0–4·0	Kehoe *et al.* (1940b)
Carrots	Brit. Columbia	2·0–4·0	Warren and Delavault (1962)
Cauliflower	U.S.A.	0	Kehoe *et al.* (1933c)
Cauliflower, leaves organically grown	U.S.A.	0·09	Schroeder and Balassa (1961)
Cauliflower	India	0·2	Bagchi *et al.* (1940)
Celery, green	U.S.A.	0·10	Schroeder and Balassa (1961)
Chicory, fresh	U.S.A.	0·81	Schroeder and Balassa (1961)
Escarole, fresh	U.S.A.	0·27	Schroeder and Balassa (1961)

Item	Country of Origin	Lead Content ppm	Authors
Vegetables (*contd.*)			
Kale, organically grown	U.S.A.	1·26	Schroeder and Balassa (1961)
Leeks		0·04–0·07	Min. of Agriculture (1972)
Leek-stem		0·7	Warren and Delavault (1962)
Lettuce	U.S.A.	0	Kehoe *et al.* (1933c)
Lettuce	India	0	Bagchi *et al.* (1940)
Lettuce, commercial	U.S.A.	0·03	Schroeder and Balassa (1961)
Lettuce	Brit. Columbia	1·0–9·0	Warren and Delavault (1962)
Lettuce, organically grown	U.S.A.	1·26	Schroeder and Balassa (1961)
Onions		<0·01–0·38	Min. of Agriculture (1972)
Onion, root	Brit. Columbia	1·0–4·0	Warren and Delavault (1962)
Peas, split, dried	U.S.A.	0	Schroeder and Balassa (1961)
Peas, canned		0–0·8	Monier-Williams (1938)
Peas, frozen		0·01–0·04	Min. of Agriculture (1972)
Peas, frozen and fresh	U.S.A.	0·02	Schroeder and Balassa (1961)
Peas	U.S.A.	0·03	Kehoe *et al.* (1940b)
Peas, fresh		0·2	Monier-Williams (1938)
Potatoes		<0·01–0·14	Min. of Agriculture (1972)
Potatoes, raw	U.S.A.	0·12	Schroeder and Balassa (1961)
Potato, tuber		0·3–1·0	Warren and Delavault (1962)
Potato, tuber	Brit. Columbia	0·40–12·0	Warren and Delavault (1962)
Radish	India	0	Bagchi *et al.* (1940)
Radish	Mexico	0·2	Kehoe *et al.* (1940b)
Soya bean	India	0	Bagchi *et al.* (1940)
Spinach	U.S.A.	0	Kehoe *et al.* (1933c)
Spinach, frozen		0·01–0·04	Min of Agriculture (1972).
Spinach	U.S.A.	0·16	Schroeder and Balassa (1961)
Swedes		<0·01–0·05	Min. of Agriculture (1972)
Watercress		0·08–0·38	Min. of Agriculture (1972)
Green vegetables		0·24	Tolan and Elton (1972)
Root vegetables		0·20	Tolan and Elton (1972)

Fruit

Apples, whole fruit		<0·01–0·16	Min. of Agriculture (1972)
Apples, skin		<0·01–0·24	Min. of Agriculture (1972)

Item	Country of Origin	Lead Content ppm	Authors
Fruit (*contd.*)			
Apples	U.S.A.	0·12	Kehoe *et al.* (1940b)
Apples	U.S.A.	0·30	Kehoe *et al.* (1933c)
Apples		0·3	Monier-Williams (1938)
Apples	India	0·3	Bagchi *et al.* (1940)
Apples	U.S.A.	0·38	Schroeder and Balassa (1961)
Bananas	U.S.A.	0	Kehoe *et al.* (1933c)
Cherries	U.S.A.	0·12	Kehoe *et al.* (1940b)
Cherries		0·5	Monier-Williams (1938)
Cherries	U.S.A.	0·77	Kehoe *et al.* (1933c)
Cranberries	U.S.A.	0·09	Kehoe *et al.* (1933c)
Gooseberries		0·3	Monier-Williams (1938)
Oranges	U.S.A.	0·00–0·04	Kehoe *et al.* (1933c)
Oranges		0·5	Monier-Williams (1938)
Peaches	U.S.A.	0	Kehoe *et al.* (1933c)
Peaches	U.S.A.	0·04–0·08	Kehoe *et al.* (1940b)
Peaches		0·9	Monier-Williams (1938)
Pears	U.S.A.	0·03	Schroeder and Balassa (1961)
Pears	U.S.A.	0·18	Kehoe *et al.* (1940b)
Pears	U.S.A.	0·21	Kehoe *et al.* (1933c)
Pears, imported		0·4	Monier-Williams (1938)
Rhubarb, stalk	Brit. Columbia	0·50–2·0	Warren and Delavault (1962)
Rhubarb, stalk		2·0–4·0	Warren and Delavault (1962)
Strawberries		0·4	Monier-Williams (1938)
Tomatoes, fresh	U.S.A.	0·02	Schroeder and Balassa (1961)
Fruits and preserves		0·12	Tolan and Elton (1972)

Meat and Fish

Item	Country of Origin	Lead Content ppm	Authors
Anchovies	U.S.A.	0·87	Schroeder and Balassa (1961)
Beef, spleen	U.S.A.	0·003–0·027	Kehoe (1961a)
Beef	U.S.A.	0·003–0·63	Kehoe *et al.* (1940b)
Beef		<0·01–0·50	Min. of Agriculture (1972)
Beef, kidney	U.S.A.	0·12–0·38	Kehoe (1960)
Beef, brain	U.S.A.	0·13	Kehoe (1960)
Beef, kidney	India	0·2	Bagchi *et al.* (1940)
Beef, chuck	U.S.A.	0·20	Schroeder and Balassa (1961)
Beef, liver	U.S.A.	0·29–0·40	Kehoe *et al.* (1940b)
Beef, liver	India	0·36–0·42	Bagchi *et al.* (1940)
Beef, bone	U.S.A.	3·60	Kehoe (1960)

Item	Country of Origin	Lead Content ppm	Authors
Meat and Fish (*contd.*)			
Clams, frozen	U.S.A.	0·15	Schroeder and Balassa (1961)
Crab, canned	Japan	0·06	Schroeder and Balassa (1961)
Crab	India	0·20–0·24	Bagchi *et al.* (1940)
Crab		0·30	Monier-Williams (1938)
Frankfurters	U.S.A.	0·16–0·20	Kehoe *et al.* (1933c)
Haddock	U.S.A.	0·27	Schroeder and Balassa (1961)
Herrings, canned		0·30	Monier-Williams (1938)
Kippers	Norway	0·30	Schroeder and Balassa (1961)
Lamb, chop	U.S.A.	0·15	Schroeder and Balassa (1961)
Lobster		0	Monier-Williams (1938)
Lobster, fresh water	India	0·08	Bagchi *et al.* (1940)
Lobster	U.S.A.	2·50	Schroeder and Balassa (1961)
Oysters, canned	U.S.A.	0·13	Schroeder and Balassa (1961)
Oysters		0·2	Monier-Williams (1938)
Pork, chop	U.S.A.	0·16	Schroeder and Balassa (1961)
Sardines, canned		0·01–2·0	Min. of Agriculture (1972)
Sardines, canned	Portugal	0·75	Schroeder and Balassa (1961)
Sausage, uncooked	U.S.A.	0·27	Kehoe *et al.* (1940b)
Sausage	U.S.A.	1·60	Kehoe *et al.* (1933c)
Scallops	U.S.A.	0·87	Schroeder and Balassa (1961)
Shrimp	India	0·24	Bagchi *et al.* (1940)
Shrimp		0·3	Monier-Williams (1938)
Shrimp, frozen	U.S.A.	0·31	Schroeder and Balassa (1961)
Shrimp, fresh	U.S.A.	0·45	Schroeder and Balassa (1961)
Winkles		1·5	Monier-Williams (1938)
Fish, fresh	India	0·0–0·54	Bagchi *et al.* (1940)
Fish		0·08	Tolan and Elton (1972)
Fish, freshwater		0·13–0·32	Min. of Agriculture (1972)
Fish, coastal water		<0·20–5·50	Min. of Agriculture (1972)
Fish, fresh	Mexico	0·24	Kehoe *et al.* (1933c)
Fish, middle-distance waters		<0·50–2·0	Min. of Agriculture (1972)
Fish, distant waters		0·5–1·0	Min. of Agriculture (1972)
Shellfish		<0·10–7·20	Min. of Agriculture (1972)
Meat, unspecified	U.S.A.	0·00–0·63	Kehoe *et al.* (1933c)
Meat and Fish		0·17	Tolan and Elton (1972)

Item	Country of Origin	Lead Content ppm	Authors
Eggs and Poultry			
Chicken	India	0·00–0·02	Bagchi *et al.* (1940)
Eggs, ducks	India	0·28–0·30	Bagchi *et al.* (1940)
Eggs		0	Monier-Williams (1938)
Eggs	U.S.A.	0·00–0·11	Kehoe *et al.* (1933c)
Eggs	U.S.A.	0·003–0·12	Kehoe *et al.* (1940b)
Eggs		<0·01–0·10	Min. of Agriculture (1972)
Eggs	India	0·24–0·25	Bagchi *et al.* (1940)
Eggs, turkeys	U.S.A.	0·02	Kehoe (1961a)
Drinks and Beverages[a]			
Beer	U.S.A.	0·01–0·29	Kehoe *et al.* (1940b)
Beer, canned	U.S.A.	0·04	Schroeder and Balassa (1961)
Brandy	India	0·05–0·06	Bagchi *et al.* (1940)
Cider	U.S.A.	0·09	Schroeder and Balassa (1961)
Gin	India	0	Bagchi *et al.* (1940)
Ginger ale	U.S.A.	0·01	Schroeder and Balassa (1961)
Lemonade	India	0·004	Bagchi *et al.* (1940)
Milk, buffalo	India	0	Bagchi *et al* (1940)
Milk, cow	India	0	Bagchi *et al.* (1940)
Milk, cow	U.S.A.	0	Schroeder and Balassa (1961)
Milk, cow	U.S.A.	0·02–0·04	Kehoe *et al.* (1940b)
Milk, cow		0·03[b]	Min. of Agriculture (1972)
Milk, cow	Italy	0·23	Lanzola *et al.* (1972)
Milk, human	U.S.A.	0·0–0·10	Kehoe *et al.* (1933c)
Milk, human	India	0·0–0·17	Bagchi *et al.* (1940)
Rum	India	0·024–0·057	Bagchi *et al.* (1940)
Soda	India	0·004	Bagchi *et al.* (1940)
Stout		0	Monier-Williams (1938)
Vinegar	U.S.A.	0·10	Schroeder and Balassa (1961)
Whisky	India	0·027	Bagchi *et al.* (1940)
Wine, red	U.S.A.	0·05	Schroeder and Balassa (1961)
Wine	U.S.A.	0·05–1·51	Kehoe *et al.* (1940b)

[a] Lead concentration in mg/litre
[b] Lead concentration in mg/kg

Item	Country of Origin	Lead Content ppm	Authors
Baby Foods			
Flours	Italy	0·0–2·4	Lanzola *et al.* (1972)
Dessert foods, in jars		<0·01–0·11	Min. of Agriculture (1972)

Item	Country of Origin	Lead Content ppm	Authors
Baby Foods (*contd.*)			
Dried milk		<0·01–0·18	Min. of Agriculture (1972)
Dried cereal		<0·01–0·26	Min. of Agriculture (1972)
Savour foods, in jars		<0·01–0·27	Min. of Agriculture (1972)
Dessert foods, canned		0·01–0·70	Min. of Agriculture (1972)
Savoury foods, canned		0·03–1·10	Min. of Agriculture (1972)
Fruit juices	Italy	<0·1–0·4	Lanzola *et al.* (1972)
Strained fruit	Italy	<0·1–2·0	Lanzola *et al.* (1972)
Strained meat	Italy	0·35–0·75	Lanzola *et al.* (1972)
Formula milk	Italy	1·5–2·4	Lanzola *et al.* (1972)

References

Afonova, V. N. (1960), *Sbornik Nauchnykh Trudov Ryazanski Meditsinss Institut* **12,** 129.

Aitcheson, L. (1960). "A History of Metals" 2 Vols, McDonald and Evans, London.

Akelaitis, A. J. (1941). *Journal of Nervous and Mental Diseases* **93,** 313.

Albahary, C. (1964). *Archives des Maladies Professionelles de Médecine du Travail et de Sécurité Sociale* **25,** 495.

Albahary, C. (1972). *Journal of the American Medical Association* **52,** 367.

Albahary, C., Truhaut, R. and Boudène, C. (1958). *Archives des Maladies Professionelles de Médecine du Travail et de Sécurité Sociale* **19,** 121.

Albahary, C., Richet, G. and Guillaume, J. (1965). *Archives des Maladies Professionelles de Médecine du Travail et de Sécurité Social* **26,** 5.

Aldanazarov, A. T., Aitbaev, T. K. and Kutyrkina, N. A. (1963). *Izvestia Akademii Nauk Kazakhskoĭ SSR, Series Med. Nauk.* **2,** 48.

Aldridge, W. N., Cremer, J. E. and Threfall, C. J. (1962). *Biochemical Pharmacology* **11,** 835.

Alexander, E. (1909). *Ophthalmologica* **5,** 634.

Alexander, F. A. and Delves, H. T. (1972). *Archives of Disease in Childhood* **47,** 446.

Alexander, F. A., Delves, H. T. and Clayton, B. E. (1972). International Symposium, Environmental Health Aspects of Lead, Amsterdam, Paper 30.

Allcroft, R. (1950). *Journal of Comparative Pathology and Therapeutics* **60,** 190.

Allcroft, R. and Blaxter, K. L. (1950). *Journal of Comparative Pathology and Therapeutics* **60,** 209.

Allen, D. W. and Jandl, J. H. (1960). *Blood* **15,** 71.

Allen-Price, E. D. (1960). *Lancet* **1,** 1235.

Allt, G. and Cavanagh, J. B. (1969). *Brain* **92,** 452.

American Academy of Pediatrics (1969). *Pediatrics*, **44,** 291

Ambrosi, L. (1962). *Folia Medica (Napoli)* **45,** 404.

Amphlett-Williams, H. (1972). *Royal Society of Health Journal* **92,** 225.

Anderson, T. W., Le Riche, W. H. and MacKay, J. S. (1969). *New England Journal of Medicine* **280,** 805.

Andres, K. H. (1961). *Zeitschrift für Zellforschung und Mikroskopische Anatomie* **55,** 49.

Andres, K. H. (1963). *Zeitschrift für Zellforschung und Mikroskopische Anatomie* **61,** 1.

Andrews, R. and Longcore, J. R. (1969), *Transactions of the 34th North American Wildlife and Natural Resources Conference, Washington,* 337.

Angevine, J. M., Kappas, A., De Gowin, R. L. and Spargo, B. H. (1962). *Archives of Pathology,* **73,** 486.

Angle, C. R. and McIntyre, M. S. (1964). *American Journal of Diseases of Children* **108,** 436.

Antal, A., Timaru, J., Muncaci, E., Ardevan, E., Ionescu, A. and Sandulache, L. (1968). *Atmospheric Environment* **2,** 383.
Aran, F. A. (1850). *Archives Génerales de Médecine* **24,** 4; 172.
Ardelean, I., Gontzea, J., Sutescu, P., Vintica, P. and Vaida, I. (1955). *Buletin Stiintific, Sectia de Stiinte Medicale* **7,** 339.
Ashby, W. (1921). *Journal of Experimental Medicine* **34,** 127.
Atkins, P. R. and Kruger, P. (1968). *Technical Report No 98, Department of Civil Engineering, Stanford Research Institute, California.*
Aub, J. C. and Reznikoff, P. (1924). *Journal of Experimental Medicine* **40,** 189.
Aub, J. C., Fairhall, L. T., Minot, A. and Reznikoff, P. (1925). *Medicine* **4,** 1.
Aub, J. C., Fairhall, L. T., Minot, A. and Reznikoff, P. (1926). "Lead Poisoning." Williams and Wilkins, Baltimore.
Ault, W. V., Senechal, R. G. and Erlebach, W. E. (1970). *Environmental Science and Technology* **4,** 305.
Azar, A., Snee, R. D. and Habibi, K. (1972). International Symposium, Environmental Health Aspects of Lead, Amsterdam, Paper 55.
Bacon, A. P. C., Froome, K., Gent, A. E., Cooke, T. K. and Sowerby, P. (1967). *Lancet* **1,** 264.
Baernstein, H. D. and Grand, J. A. (1942). *Journal of Pharmacology and Experimental Therapeutics* **74,** 18.
Bagchi, K. N., Ganguly, H. D. and Sirdar, J. N. (1940). *Indian Journal of Medical Research* **27,** 777.
Bagley, G. E., Locke, L. N. and Nightingale, G. T. (1967). *Avian Diseases* **11,** 601.
Baker, G. (1767). "An Essay Concerning the Cause of the Endemial Colic of Devonshire." T. Cadell, London.
Baker, G. (1768). *Medical Transactions of the College of Physicians, London* **1,** 319.
Baker, J. B. E. (1960). *Pharmacological Reviews* **12,** 37.
Balbo, W. and Marucci, V. (1962). *Zacchia* **25,** 419.
Balbo, W., Gualdi, G. and Marucci, V. (1965). *Folia Medica (Napoli)* **48,** 544.
Ball, G. V. and Sorensen, L. B. (1969). *New England Journal of Medicine* **280,** 1199.
Banciu, T. and Petrovici, A. (1968). *Acta Gastro-enterologica Belgica* **31,** 693.
Barltrop, D. (1969). *In* "Mineral Metabolism in Paediatrics" (D. Barltrop and W. L. Burland, eds.) p. 135. Blackwell, Oxford.
Barnes, J. R., Smith, P. E. and Drummond, C. M. (1972). *Archives of Environmental Health* **25,** 450.
Baron, J. (1954). Thesis, Lyons.
Barry, P. S. I. (1972). International Symposium, Environmental Health Aspects of Lead, Amsterdam, Paper 38.
Barry, P. S. I. and Harrison, G. F. (1972). *Petroleum Review* **26,** 311.
Barry, P. S. I. and Mossman, D. B. (1970). *British Journal of Industrial Medicine* **27,** 339.
Barry, P. S. I. and Turner, D. (1964). *Lancet* **1,** 1275.
Bashour, F. A. (1954). *Journal of Laboratory and Clinical Medicine* **44,** 764.
Bastenier, H., Deslypère, P. and Mme de Graef-Millet (1957). *Proceedings 12th International Congress on Occupational Health, Helsinki,* Vol. III, 243.
Baydens, M. R. (1957). *Bulletin de l'Académie Royale de Médecine de Belgique* **22,** 293.
Bazell, R. J. (1971). *Science* **173,** 130.
Beattie, A. D., Dagg, J. H., Goldberg, A., Wang, I. and Ronald, J. (1972a). *British Medical Journal* **2,** 488.
Beattie, A. D., Moore, W. R., Devenay, W. T., Miller, A. R. and Goldberg, A. (1972b). *British Medical Journal* **2,** 491.

Beattie, A. D., Moore, M. R. and Goldberg, A. (1972c). *Lancet* **2,** 12.
Beaver, D. L. (1961). *American Journal of Pathology* **39,** 195.
Beck, E., Lanini, G. and Béraud, T. (1955). *Helvetica Medica Acta* **22,** 442.
Becker, R. O., Spadaro, J. A. and Berg, E. W. (1968). *Journal of Bone and Joint Surgery* **A50,** 326.
Behrens, B. and Baumann, A. (1933–1934). *Zeitschrift für die Gesamte Experimentelle Medizin* **92,** 251.
Belknap, E. L. (1936). *Journal of Industrial Hygiene* **18,** 380.
Belknap, E. L. (1952). *Industrial Medicine* **21,** 305.
Bell, W. B. (1924). *Lancet* **1,** 268.
Bell, W. B., Williams, W. R. and Cunningham, L. (1925). *Lancet* **2,** 793.
Belli, R., Maggio, M. and Arciello, G. (1955). *Folia Medica (Napoli)* **38,** 790.
Bénard, H., Rambert, P., Gajdos, A., Gajdos-Török, A. and Malvezin, M. (1950). *Bulletin et Mémoires de la Société de Médecine de Paris* **21/22,** 1120.
Berdyev, Kh. B., Pavlovich, N. V. and Tuzhilina, A. A. (1967). *Gigiena i Sanitaria* **32,** 6; 96.
Berg, J. M. and Zappella, M. (1964). *Journal of Mental Deficiency Research* **8,** 44.
Bergamini, V. and Sibour, F. (1960). *Rivista di Patologia Nervosa e Mentale* **81,** 415.
Bergner, K. G. and Miethke, H. (1964). *Zeitschrift für Lebensmitteluntersuchung und -Forschung* **125,** 406.
Beritić, T. (1963). *British Journal of Haematology* **9,** 185.
Beritić, T. (1971). *Archives of Environmental Health* **23,** 289.
Beritić, T. and Stahuljak, D. (1961). *Lancet* **1,** 669.
Berk, P. D., Tschudy, D. P., Shepley, L. A., Waggoner, J. G. and Berlin, N. I. (1970). *American Journal of Medicine* **48,** 137.
Berlin, A., del Castilho, P. and Smeets, J. (1972). International Symposium, Environmental Health Aspects of Lead, Amsterdam, Paper 92.
Berlin, N. I., Waldmann, T.A. and Weissman, S. M. (1959). *Physiological Reviews* **39,** 577.
Bersin, T. (1958). *Vitalstoffe* **3,** 160.
Bertrand, G. and Okada, Y. (1933). *Chemical Abstracts* **27,** 3022.
Bessis, M. (1958). *Bulletin de l'Académie Nationale de Médecine, Paris* **142,** 629.
Bessis, M. and Breton-Gorius, J. (1957a). *Compte rendu hebdomadaire des Séances de l'Académie des Sciences (Paris)* **244,** 2846.
Bessis, M. and Breton-Gorius, J. (1957b). *Revue d'Hématologie* **12,** 43.
Bessis, M. and Breton-Gorius, J. (1957c). *Semaine des Hôpitaux de Paris (Path. et Biol.)* **33,** 411.
Bessis, M. and Breton-Gorius, J. (1957d). *Compte rendu des Séances de la Société de Biologie (Paris)* **151,** 275.
Bessis, M. and Breton-Gorius, J. (1959). *Blood* **14,** 423.
Bessis, M. and Jensen, W. N. (1965). *British Journal of Haematology* **11,** 49.
Bessman, S. P., Reid, H. and Rubin, M. (1952). *Medical Annals of the District of Columbia* **21,** 312.
Betts, P. R., Astley, R. and Raine, D. N. (1973). *British Medical Journal* **1,** 402.
Biersteker, K. (1967). *Tijdschrift voor Sociale Geneeskunde* **45,** 658.
Bingham, E., Pfitzer, E. A., Barkley, W. and Radford, E. P. (1968). *Science* **162,** 1297.
Biondi, S. (1955). *Folia Medica (Napoli)* **38,** 133.
Biorck, G., Böström, H. and Widstrom, A. (1965). *Acta Medica Scandinavica* **178,** 239.
Black, S. C. (1962). *Archives of Environmental Health* **5,** 423.
Blackman, S. S. (1936). *Bulletin of the Johns Hopkins Hospital* **58,** 384.
Blackmore, D. R. (1972). *Petroleum Review* **26,** 169.

Blanksma, L. A., Sachs, H. K., Murray, E. F. and O'Connell, M. J. (1969). *Pediatrics* **44,** 661.
Blaxter, K. L. (1950). *Journal of Comparative Pathology and Therapeutics* **60,** 140.
Blaxter, K. L. and Cowie, A. T. (1946). *Nature* **157,** 588.
Blemel, K. G. (1967). *Archives of Environmental Health* **14,** 594.
Blokker, P. C. (1972). *Atmospheric Environment* **6,** 1.
Blumenthal, S., Davidow, B., Harris, D. and Oliver-Smith, F. (1972). *American Journal of Public Health* **62,** 1060.
Boddy, J. H. (1972). *Petroleum Review* **26,** 284.
Bolanowska, W. (1968). *British Journal of Industrial Medicine* **25,** 203.
Bolanowska, W., Pitrowski, J. and Trojanowska, B. (1964). *Proceedings 14th International Congress of Occupational Health, Madrid,* p. 420.
Bonsignore, D. (1966). *Medicina del Lavoro* **57,** 647.
Bonsignore, D., Calissano, P. and Cartasegna, C. (1965). *Medicina del Lavoro* **56,** 199.
Booker, D. V., Chamberlain, A. C., Newton, D. and Scott, A. N. B. (1969). *British Journal of Radiology* **42,** 457.
Borsook, H., Fischer, E. F. and Keighley, G. (1957). *Journal of Biological Chemistry* **229,** 1059.
Boström, H. and Webster, P. O. (1967). *Acta Medica Scandinavica* **181,** 465.
Boulakia, J. D. C. (1972). *American Journal of Archaeology* **76,** 139.
Boulding, J. E. and Baker, R. A. (1957). *Lancet* **2,** 985.
Bowman, H. R., Conway, J. G. and Asaro, F. (1972). *Environmental Science and Technology* **6,** 558.
Boyadjiev, V., Chalatcheva, L. and Nokolova, P. (1968). *Archiv für Gewerbepathologie und Gewerbehygiene* **24,** 299.
Boyett, J. D. and Butterworth, C. E. (1962). *American Journal of Medicine* **32,** 884.
Boyett, J. D., Pitman, J. A. and Butterworth, C. E. (1960). *Clinical Research* **8,** 52.
Boyland, E., Dukes, C. E., Grover, P. L. and Mitchley, B. C. V. (1962). *British Journal of Cancer* **16,** 283.
Bradley, J. E. and Baumgartner, R. J. (1958). *Journal of Pediatrics* **53,** 311.
Bradley, J. E., Powell, A. E., Niermann, W., McGrady, K. R. and Kaplan, E. (1956). *Journal of Pediatrics* **49,** 1.
Braun, H. A., Lusky, L. M. and Calvery, H. O. (1946). *Journal of Pharmacology and Experimental Therapeutics* **87,** 119.
Breinl, A. and Young, W. J. (1914). *Annals of Tropical Medicine and Parasitology* **8,** 575.
Brief, R. S. (1962). *Archives of Environmental Health* **5,** 527.
Brieger, H. (1960). *Archives of Environmental Health* **1,** 271.
Brigatti, L., Parigi, A. and Varetto, L. (1962). *Médecine Sociale et Professionelle* **53,** 1268.
Brookfield, R. W. (1928). *Journal of Pathology and Bacteriology* **31,** 277.
Brooks, A. L. (1951). *Industrial Medicine* **20,** 390.
Brose, L. D. (1915). *Archives of Ophthalmology* **44,** 26.
Brown, A. (1946). *Quarterly Journal of Medicine* **15,** 77.
Brown, A. and Tompsett, S. L. (1945). *British Medical Journal* **2,** 764.
Brown, J. S. (1962). *Economic Geology* **57,** 673.
Brown, S., Dragann, N. and Vogel, W. H. (1971). *Archives of Environmental Health* **22,** 370.
de Bruin, A. (1968). *Medicina del Lavoro* **59,** 411.
de Bruin, A. (1971). *Archives of Environmental Health* **23,** 249.
de Bruin, A. and Holboom, H. (1967). *British Journal of Industrial Medicine* **24,** 203.
de Bruin, A. and Jong-Heisterkamp, G. T. (1968). *Annales de Biologie Clinique* **26,** 717.

Bryce-Smith, D. (1971a). *Chemistry in Britain* **7,** 54.
Bryce-Smith, D. (1971b). *Chemistry in Britain* **7,** 284.
Bryce-Smith, D. (1971c). *Biologist* **18,** 52.
Bryce-Smith, D. (1972a). *Chemistry in Britain* **8,** 240.
Bryce-Smith, D. (1972b). *Lancet* **2,** 817.
Bryce-Smith, D. (1973). *Journal of the Royal Society of Arts* **121,** 120.
Buck, J. S. and Kumro, D. M. (1930). *Journal of Pharmacology and Experimental Therapeutics* **38,** 161.
Buck, W. B. (1970). *Journal of the American Veterinary Medical Association* **156,** 1468.
Buckup, H. and Mappes, R. (1962). *Zentralblatt für Arbeitsmedizin und Arbeitsschutz* **12,** 293.
Buczkowski, M. (1964). *Archiv für Gewerbepathologie und Gewerbehygiene* **20,** 537.
Bugler, J. and Doyle, C. (1972). *The Observer*, 31 December.
Bugler, J. and Doyle, C. (1973). *The Observer*, 7 January.
Bullock, J. and Lewis, W. M. (1968). *Atmospheric Environment* **2,** 517.
Bullock, J. D., Wey, R. J., Zaia, J. A., Zarembock, I. and Schroeder, H. A. (1966). *Archives of Environmental Health* **13,** 21.
Bulpitt, C. J. (1972). *Lancet* **2,** 1144.
Bunge, R. P., Bunge, M. P. and Ris, H. (1960). *Journal of Biophysical and Biochemical Cytology* **7,** 685.
de la Burde, B. (1972). *Journal of Pediatrics* **80,** 629.
Burton, H. (1840). *Medico-Chirurgical Transactions* **23,** 63.
Burton, W. M. and Stewart, N. G. (1960). *Nature* **186,** 584.
Butt, E. M., Peason, H. E. and Simonsen, D. G. (1952). *Proceedings of the Society for Experimental Biology and Medicine* **79,** 247.
Byers, R. K. (1959). *Pediatrics* **23,** 585.
Byers, R. K. and Lord, E. (1943). *American Journal of Diseases of Children* **66,** 471.
Byers, R. K. and Maloof, C. C. (1954). *American Journal of Diseases of Children* **87,** 559.
Caccuri, S. and Pecora, L. (1972). International Symposium, Environmental Health Aspects of Lead, Amsterdam, Paper 75.
Caffey, J. (1938). *American Journal of Diseases of Children* **55,** 798.
Calhoun, J. A., McLean, R., Hudson, J. C. and Aub, J. C. (1954). *Archives of Industrial Hygiene* **9,** 9.
California Public Health Department (1967). "Lead in the Environment and its Effects on Humans."
Calingaert, G., Shapiro, H., Dykstra, F. J. and Hess, L. (1948). *Journal of the American Chemical Society* **16,** 191.
Camba, R., Dianzani, M. A. and Montaldo, S. (1963). *Rassegna Medica Sarda* **65,** 591.
Campbell, A. M. G. (1955). *Lancet* **2,** 376.
Campbell, A. M. G. and Williams, E. R. (1968). *British Medical Journal* **4,** 582.
Campbell, A. M. G., Herdan, F., Tatlow, W. F. T. and Whittle, E. G. (1950). *Brain* **73,** 52.
Campbell, A. M. G., Williams, E. R. and Barltrop, D. (1970). *Journal of Neurology, Neurosurgery and Psychiatry* **33,** 877.
Cannon, H. L. and Bowles, J. M. (1962). *Science* **137,** 765.
Cantarow, A. and Trumper, M. (1944). "Lead Poisoning." Williams and Wilkins, Baltimore.
Carpenter, K. E. (1924). *Annals of Applied Biology* **11,** 1.
Carpenter, K. E. (1925). *Annals of Applied Biology* **12,** 1.
Carpenter, K. E. (1926). *Annals of Applied Biology* **13,** 395.

Carr, T. E. F., Nolan, J. and Duraković, A. (1969). *Nature* **224,** 115.
Cassells, D. A. K. and Dodds, E. C. (1946). *British Medical Journal* **2,** 681.
Castellino, N. and Aloj, S. (1964). *British Journal of Industrial Medicine* **21,** 308.
Castellino, N. and Aloj, S. (1969). *British Journal of Industrial Medicine* **26,** 139.
Castellino, N., Rossi, A. and Molé, R. (1963). *British Journal of Industrial Medicine* **20,** 63.
Castellino, N., Lamanna, P. and Grieco, B. (1965). *Folia Medica (Napoli)* **48,** 601.
Castellino, N., Lamanna, P. and Grieco, B. (1966). *British Journal of Industrial Medicine* **23,** 237.
Casula, D., Cherchi, P., Piredda, S. and Spinnazola, A. (1959). *Rassegna Medica Sarda* **61,** 847.
Casula, D., Cherchi, P. and Spinnazola, A. (1960a). *Rassegna Italiana di Gastro-Enterologia*, **6,** 639.
Casula, D., Cherchi, P. and Spinnazola, A. (1960b). *Rassegna Medica Sarda* **62,** 703.
Cataldi, R. and Odaglia, G. (1958). *Archives des Maladies Professionelles de Médecine du Travail et de Sécurité Sociale* **19,** 467.
Catton, M. J., Harrison, M. J. G., Fullerton, P. M. and Kazantzis, G. (1970). *British Medical Journal* **2,** 80.
Cavanagh, J. B. and Jacobs, J. M. (1964). *British Journal of Experimental Pathology* **45,** 309.
Cerquiglini-Monteriolo, S. and Funiciello, R. (1972). International Symposium, Environmental Health Aspects of Lead, Amsterdam, Paper 86.
Cervetti, S. and Casucci, G. (1960). *Lavoro Umano* **12,** 452.
Challop, R., McCabe, E. and Reece, R. (1972). *American Journal of Public Health* **62,** 655.
Chamberlain, G. T. (1959). *East African Agricultural Journal* **25,** 121.
Chamberlain, M. J. and Massey, P. M. O. (1972). *British Journal of Industrial Medicine,* **29,** 458.
Charache, S. and Weatherall, D. J. (1966). *Blood* **28,** 377.
Chia, B. L., Leng, C. K., Hsii, F. P., Yap, M. H. L. and Lee, Y. K. (1973). *British Medical Journal* **1,** 354.
Chiesura, P. and Brugnone, F. (1963). *Medicina del Lavoro* **54,** 88.
Chiodi, H. and Sammartino, R. A. (1947). *Nature* **160,** 680.
Chisholm, J. J. (1964). *Journal of Pediatrics* **64,** 174.
Chisholm, J. J. (1965). *Developmental Medicine and Child Neurology* **7,** 529.
Chisholm, J. J. (1968). *Journal of Pediatrics* **73,** 1.
Chisholm, J. J. (1970). *Pediatric Clinics of North America* **17,** 591.
Chisholm, J. J. (1972). *Journal of Pediatrics* **80,** 628.
Chisholm, J. J. and Harrison, H. E. (1956). *Pediatrics* **18,** 943.
Chisholm, J. J. and Leahy, N. B. (1962). *Journal of Pediatrics* **60,** 1.
Chisholm, J. J., Harrison, H. C., Eberlein, W. R. and Harrison, H. E. (1955). *American Journal of Diseases of Children* **89,** 159.
Choi, H. (1963). *Bulletin of Korean Industrial Medicine* **2,** 23.
Choie, D. D. and Richter, G. W. (1972a). *American Journal of Pathology* **66,** 265.
Choie, D. D. and Richter, G. W. (1972b). *Science* **177,** 1194.
Cholak, J., Schafer, L. J. and Sterling, T. D. (1961). *Journal of the Air Pollution Control Association,* **11,** 281.
Cholak, J., Schafer, L. J. and Yeager, D. (1968). *American Industrial Hygiene Association Journal* **29,** 562.
Chow, T. J. (1971). *In* "Proceedings of the Second International Clear Air Congress" (H. M. England and W. T. Beery, eds.) p. 348. Academic Press, New York.

Chow, T. J. and Earl, J. L. (1970). *Science* **169,** 577.
Chow, T. J. and Johnstone, M. S. (1965). *Science* **147,** 502.
Chow, T. J. and Patterson, C. C. (1966). *Earth and Planet Science Letters* **1,** 397.
Chow, T. J., Earl, J. L. and Bennett, C. F. (1969). *Environmental Science and Technology* **3,** 737.
Chow, T. J., Earl, J. L. and Snyder, C. B. (1972). *Science* **178,** 401.
Christian, J. R., Celewycz, B. S. and Andelmann, S. L. (1964). *American Journal of Public Health* **54,** 1241.
Cikrt, M. (1972). *British Journal of Industrial Medicine* **29,** 74.
Civil Aviation Authority (1972). Airworthiness Notice No 70, 25 September.
Clark, K. G. A. (1972). *Lancet* **2,** 662.
Clarkson, T. W. and Kench, J. E. (1956). *Biochemical Journal* **62,** 361.
Clarkson, T. W. and Kench, J. E. (1958). *Biochemical Journal* **69,** 432.
Clegg, F. G. and Rylands, J. M. (1966). *Journal of Comparative Pathology and Therapeutics* **76,** 15.
Cline, M. J. and Berlin, N. I. (1963a). *Blood* **22,** 459.
Cline, M. J. and Berlin, N. I. (1963b). *Journal of Laboratory and Clinical Medicine* **61,** 249.
Cogbill, E. C. and Hobbs, M. E. (1957). *Tobacco Science*, 10 May.
Cohen, G. J. and Ahrens, W. E. (1959). *Journal of Pediatrics* **54,** 271.
Cohen, S., Sweet, A. Y., Mautner, W., Churg, J. and Grishman, E. (1960). *American Journal of Diseases of Children* **100,** 559.
Colucci, J. M., Begeman, C. R. and Kumler, K. (1969). *Journal of the Air Pollution Control Association* **19,** 225.
Combrisson, A., Desoille, H. and Albahary, C. (1964). *Proceedings of the 14th International Congress on Occupational Health, Madrid*, Vol. 2, 755.
Committee on Ethyl Petrol (1930). "Final Report," H.M.S.O., London.
Conway, N. (1940). *Industrial Medicine* **9,** 471.
Coombes, A. H. (1972). "Lead in Paints." Report of the City Analyst to the Health Committee, City of Birmingham.
Cooper, C. (1947). *American Journal of Roentgenology* **58,** 129.
Cooper, R. G., Webster, L. T. and Harris, J. W. (1963). *Journal of Clinical Investigation* **42,** 926.
Corsi, G. C. and Galzigna, L. (1963). *Lavoro Umano* **15,** 364.
Craig, P. P. (1970). "Lead in the Biosphere—A Case Study in Unnecessary Industrial Pollution." Brookhaven National Laboratory, Upton, N.Y.
Cramér, K. (1966). *Acta Medica Scandinavica, Suppl.* **445,** 56.
Cramér, K. and Selander, S. (1965). *British Journal of Industrial Medicine* **22,** 311.
Crawford, M. D. and Crawford, T. (1969). *Lancet* **1,** 699.
Crawford, M. D. and Morris, J. N. (1967). *Lancet* **2,** 1087.
Crawford, M. D., Gardner, M. J. and Morris, J. N. (1968). *Lancet* **1,** 827.
Crawford, M. D., Gardner, M. J. and Sedgwick, P. A. (1972), *Lancet* **1,** 988.
Crawford, T. and Crawford, M. D. (1967). *Lancet* **1,** 229.
Cremer, J. E. (1959). *British Journal of Industrial Medicine* **16,** 191.
Cremer, J. E. (1962a). *Journal of Neurochemistry* **9,** 289.
Cremer, J. E. (1962b). *Nature* **195,** 607.
Cremer, J. E. and Callaway, S. (1961). *British Journal of Industrial Medicine* **18,** 277.
Crepet, M., Gobbato, F., Martino, P. and Siravusa, F. (1956). *Minerva Nefrologica* **3,** 69.
Crepet, M., Rubino, G. and Gobbato, F. (1956). *Proceedings 21st Congress Nationale di Medicina del Lavoro, Merano*, p. 1.

Crutcher, J. C. (1963). *Archives of Internal Medicine* **59,** 707.
Csillik, B. (1965). "Functional Structure of the Postsynaptic Membrane in the Myoneural Junction." Akadémiai Kiadó, Budapest.
Cubasik, N. P. and Volasin, M. T. (1972). *Clinical Chemistry* **18,** 1415.
Cumings, J. N (1959). "Heavy Metals and the Brain." C. C. Thomas, Springfield.
Cund, F. R. N. and Murray, J. R. (1954). *Journal of the American Chemical Society* **76,** 187.
Currier, R. D. and Haerer, A. F. (1968). *Archives of Environmental Health* **17,** 712.
Dagg, J. H., Goldberg, A., Lochhead, A. and Smith, J. A. (1965). *Quarterly Journal of Medicine* **34,** 163.
Daines, R. H., Motto, H. L. and Chilko, D. M. (1970). *Environmental Science and Technology* **4,** 318.
Daines, R. H., Smith, D. W., Feliciano, A. and Trout, J. R. (1972). *Industrial Medicine* **41,** 26.
Dalldorf, G. and Williams, R. R. (1945). *Science* **102,** 668.
Dallenbach, F. (1964). *Virchows Archiv für Pathologische Anatomie und Physiologie und für Klinische Medizin* **338,** 91.
Danieli, G., Gajdos-Török, M. and Gajdos, A. (1961). *Pathologie et Biologie* **9,** 1481.
Danielson, L. (1969). Bulletin No. 6, Ecological Research Committee, Swedish Natural Science Research Council, Stockholm.
Dannenberg, A. M., Widerman, A. H. and Friedmann, P. S. (1940). *Journal of the American Medical Association* **114,**, 1439.
Dautrebande, L. and Walkenhorst, W. (1961). *In* "Inhaled Particles and Vapours" (C. N. Davies ed.) p. 117. Pergamon Press, London,
David, A. (1963). *Časopis Lékaru Českých* **102,** 69.
David, O., Clark, J. and Voeller, K. (1972). *Lancet* **2,** 900.
Davis, J. R., Abrahams, R. H., Fishbein, W. I. and Fabrega, E. A. (1968). *Archives of Environmental Health* **17,** 164.
Davis, J. R. and Andelman, S. L. (1967). *Archives of Environmental Health* **15,** 53.
Dawson, E. B., Cravy, W. D., Clark, R. R. and McGavity, W. J. (1965). *American Journal of Obstetrics and Gynecology* **103,** 253.
Dean, G. (1971). "The Porphyrias," Pitman Medical, London.
Delwaide, P. J. and Chantraine, A. (1965). *Proceedings of the 6th International Congress on Electroencephology and Clinical Neurophysiology, Vienna*, p. 643.
Desoille, H., Albahary, C., Truhaut, R. and Boudene, C. (1957). *Proceedings of the 12th International Congress on Occupational Health, Helsinki*, Vo. 3, p. 287.
Desoille, H., Philbert, M. and Albahary, C. (1970). *Archives des Maladies Professionelles de Médecine du Travail et de Sécurité Sociale* **31,** 221.
Detwille, S. R. and Kehoe, K. (1939). *Journal of Experimental Zoology* **81,** 415.
Devergie, A. and Hervy, O. (1838). *Annales d'Hygiène* **20,** 463.
Dingwall-Fordyce, I. and Lane, R. E. (1963). *British Journal of Industrial Medicine* **20,** 313.
Di Luzzio, N. (1972). *Chemical Engineering News*, February 28, p. 56.
Djurić, D. D., Novak, L., Milic, S. and Kalic-Filipovic, D. (1966). *Medicina del Lavoro* **57,** 161.
Doinikow, V. B. (1911). *Arbeiten über die Grosshirnrinde* **4,** 445.
Dolowitz, D., Fazekas, J. F. and Himwich, H. T. (1937). *Journal of Industrial Hygiene* **19,** 93.
Donovan, D. T., Vought, V. M. and Rakow, A. B. (1971). *Archives of Environmental Health* **23,** 111.

Dreeson, W. C., Edwards, T. I. and Reinhart, W. H. (1941). Public Health Bulletin No. 262, Federal Security Agency, Public Health Service.
Dresel, E. I. and Falk, J. E. (1956). *Biochemical Journal* **63,** 72.
Druyan, R. and Haeger-Aronsen, B. (1964). *Scandinavian Journal of Clinical and Laboratory Investigation* **16,** 498.
Dubrovskaya, F. I. (1960). *Gigiena i Sanitariya* **25,** 4.
Dudley, H. R., Ritchie, A. C., Schilling, A. and Baker, W. H. (1955). *New England Journal of Medicine* **252,** 331.
Dunn, J. T. and Bloxham, H. C. L. (1932). *Journal of the Society of Chemical Industry* **51,** 100.
Dustin, P. (1943). *Archives de Biologie (Liége)* **55,** 475.
Dustin, P. (1944). *Archives de Biologie (Liége)* **56,** 285.
Dyck, P. J. and Gomez, M. R. (1968). *Mayo Clinic Proceedings* **43,** 280.
Eadie, G. S., Smith, W. W. and Brown, I. W. (1960). *Journal of General Physiology* **43,** 825.
Eanes, E. D. and Posner, A. S. (1967). *In* "Small Angle X-ray Scattering" (H. Baumberger ed.) p. 283. Gradon and Breach, New York.
Egan, H. (1972). *In* "Lead in the Environment" (P. Hepple ed.) p. 34. Institute of Petroleum, London.
Egli, R., Grandjean, G., Marmet, J. and Kapps, H. (1957). *Schweizerische Medizinische Wochenschrift* **87,** 1171.
Egorov, V. V., Zhigalovskaya, T. N. and Malakhov, S. G. (1970). *Journal of Geophysical Research* **75,** 3650.
Egorova, G. M., Ivanov, N. G. and Sanotskii, I. V. (1966). *Toksikologiya novykh promyshöennykh khimicheskikh veshchestv.* **8,** 33.
Eidg. Gesundheidsamt, Bern (1961). "Mitteilung aus dem Gebiete der Lebensmitteluntersuchung und Hygiene", Vol. 3.
Eldridge, W. A. (1924). Report 29, Chemical Warfare Service.
Ellis, M. M. (1937). *United States Fisheries Bulletin* **48,** 365.
Elwood, P. C., Bainton, D., Moore, F., Davies, D. F., Wakley, E. J., Langman, M. and Sweetnam, P. (1971). *British Medical Journal* **2,** 362.
Emmerson, B. T. (1963). *Australian Annals of Medicine* **12,** 310.
Emmerson, B. T. (1964). *Proceedings 2nd International Congress on Nephrology, Amsterdam*, p. 802.
Emmerson, B. T. (1965). *Australian Annals of Medicine* **14,** 295.
Emmerson, B. T. (1967). *In* "Renal Disease" (D. A. K. Black ed.), Second Edition, p. 561. Blackwell, Oxford.
Endo, R., Kohgo, T., Oyake, T., Suguwara, N., Sakamoto, T., Nakabayashi, N. and Kamada, K. (1968). *Chemical Abstracts* **69,** 89531.
Eriksen, L. (1955). *Scandinavian Journal of Clinical and Laboratory Investigation* **7,** 80.
Ettinger, M. B. (1966). "Symposium on Environmental Lead Contamination." U.S. Public Health Service Publication No. 1440, p. 21.
Evans, E. E., Norwood, W. D., Kehoe, R. A. and Machle, W. (1943). *Journal of the American Medical Association* **121,** 501.
Fairhall, L. T. and Sayers, R. R. (1940). *Public Health Bulletin (U.S.)* No. 253.
Fairley, K. D. (1934). *Medical Journal of Australia* **1,** 600.
Farkas, W. R., Hewins, S. and Welch, J.W. (1972). *Chemico-Biological Interactions* **5,** 191.
Fatzer, R. (1961). *Vitalstoffe* **5,** 26.
Fatzer, R. (1962). *Vitalstoffe* **6,** 53.
Felt, A. E. and Kerley, R. V. (1971). *Automobile Engineer* **79,** 54.

di Ferrante, E. and Bourdeau, P. (1972). International Symposium, Environmental Health Aspects of Lead, Amsterdam, Paper 33.

Ferm, V. H. (1969). *Experientia* **25,** 56.

Ferm, V. H. and Carpenter, S. J. (1967). *Experimental Molecular Pathology* **7,** 208.

Ferraro, A. and Hernandez, R. (1932). *Psychiatric Quarterly* **6,** 319.

Finner, L. L. and Calvery, H. O. (1939). *Archives of Pathology* **27,** 433.

Fisher, L. E. (1954). *Journal of the American Veterinary Medical Association* **125,** 478.

Fleisch, H., Bisaz, S. and Russel, R. (1965). *Proceedings of the Society of Experimental and Biological Medicine* **118,** 882.

Flesch, P. (1954). *In* "Physiology and Biochemistry of Skin" (S. Rothman ed.) p. 601. University of Chicago Press, Chicago.

Follis, R. H., Jackson, D., Eliot, M. M. and Park, E. A. (1943). *American Journal of Diseases of Children* **66,** 1.

Forbes, G. B. and Reina, J. C. (1972). *Journal of Nutrition* **102,** 647.

Foreman, H. (1955). *Industrial Medicine* **24,** 287.

Foreman, H. (1963). *Journal of Chronic Diseases* **16,** 319.

Foreman, H., Finnegan, C. and Lushbaugh, C. C. (1956). *Journal of the American Medical Association* **160,** 1042.

Francis, C. W., Chesters, G. and Haskin, L. A. (1970). *Environmental Science and Technology* **4,** 586.

Fratianne, R. B., Griggs, R. C. and Harris, J. W. (1959). *Clinical Research* **7,** 384.

Freeman, R. (1965). *Archives of Diseases in Childhood* **40,** 389.

Fromke, V. L., Lee, M. Y. and Watson, C. J. (1969). *Annals of Internal Medicine* **70,** 1007.

Fry, L. M. and Menon, K. K. (1962). *Science* **137,** 994.

Fullerton, J. M. (1952). *British Medical Journal* **2,** 117.

Fullerton, P. M. (1966). *Journal of Neuropathology and Experimental Neurology* **25,** 214.

Gajdos, A. and Gajdos-Török, M. (1964). *Revue Française d'Etudes Cliniques et Biologiques* **9,** 629.

Gajdos, A. and Gajdos-Török, M. (1971). *Archives of Environmental Health* **23,** 270.

Gajdos-Török, M., Gajdos, A. and Bernard, H. (1960). *Compte Rendu des Séances de la Société de Biologie* **154,** 508.

Gallé, P. and Morel-Maroger, L. (1965). *Nephron* **2,** 273.

Galzigna, L., Brugnone, F. and Corsi, G. C. (1964). *Medicina del Lavoro* **55,** 102.

Garcin, R., Lapresle, J., Fardeau, M. and de Recondo, J. (1966). *Revue Neurologique (Paris)* **115,** 917.

Garrod, A. E. (1892). *Journal of Physiology* **13,** 598.

Gartenmann, E. (1971). *Bulletin des Eidgenössischen Gesundheitsamtes* No. 3.

Gasto, B. (1959). *Medycynya Pracy.* **10,** 39.

Gattner, H. and Schrantz, G. (1964). *Deutsche Medizinische Wochenschrift* **89,** 1027.

Gayler, J. (1887). Dissertation, Tübingen.

Geleriu, R. and Strauss, H. (1972). International Symposium, Environmental Health Aspects of Lead, Amsterdam, Paper 22.

Gel'fon, I. A. and Zorina, I. A. (1964). *Gigiena Truda i Professional'nȳe Zabolevaniya* **8,** 24.

Giannattasio, R. C. (1956). *New York State Journal of Medicine* **56,** 3510.

Giannattasio, R. C., Bedo, A.V. and Pirozzi, M. J. (1952). *American Journal of Diseases of Childhood* **84,** 316.

Gibb, J. W. G. and MacMahon, J. F. (1955). *British Medical Journal* **1,** 320.

Gibbs, K. and Walshe, J. M. (1966). *Lancet* **1,** 175.

Gibson, J. and Goldberg, A. (1956). *Journal of Pathology and Bacteriology* **71,** 495.
Gibson, J. L., Love, W., Hardy, D., Bancroft, P. and Turner, A. J. (1892). *Transactions Intercolonial Medical Congress of Australia*, p. 76.
Gibson, K. D., Neuberger, A. and Scott, J. J. (1955). *Biochemical Journal* **61,** 618.
Gibson, S. L. M. and Goldberg, A. (1970). *Clinical Science* **38,** 63.
Gibson, S. L. M., Lam, C. N., McCrae, W. M. and Goldberg, A. (1967). *Archives of Disease in Childhood* **42,** 573.
Gibson, S. L. M., McKenzie, J. C. and Goldberg, A. (1968). *British Journal of Industrial Medicine* **25,** 40.
Gilfillan, S. C. (1965). *Journal of Occupational Medicine* **7,** 53.
Giménez, E. R., Vallejo, N. E., Izurieta, M. and Singerman, A. (1970). *Revista de la Associación Bioquimica Argentina* **35,** 179.
Giraud, G., Latour, H., Lévy, A., Puech, P., Olivier, G. and Hertault, J. (1959). *Montpellier Médicale* **55,** 120.
Giubileo, M. (1957). *Medicina del Lavoro* **48,** 165.
Giubileo, M. (1967). *Rivista dei Cimbustilili* **2,** 157.
Goldberg, A. (1959). *Quarterly Journal of Medicine* **28,** 183.
Goldberg, A. (1960). *Proceedings 2e Colloque International de Biologie de Saclay* p. 105.
Goldberg, A., Paton, W. D. M. and Thompson, J. W. (1954). *British Journal of Pharmacology* **9,** 91.
Goldberg, A., Ashenbrucker, H., Cartwright, G. C. and Wintrobe, M. M. (1956). *Blood* **11,** 821.
Goldblum, R. W., Derby, S. and Lerner, A. B. (1953). *Journal of Investigative Dermatology* **20,** 13.
Goldsmith, J. R. (1964). *Archives of Environmental Health* **8,** 39.
Goldsmith, J. R. (1969). *Journal of the Air Pollution Control Association* **19,** 714.
Goldsmith, J. R. (1972). *Lancet* **2,** 661.
Goldsmith, J. R. and Hexter, A. C. (1967). *Science* **158,** 132.
Goldsmith, J. R. and Hexter, A. C. (1968). *Science* **159,** 1000.
Goldwater, L. J. (1972). *Industrial Medicine* **41,** 13.
Goldwater, L. J. and Hoover, A. W. (1967). *Archives of Environmental Health* **15,** 60.
Golubovich, E. Y., Avkhimenko, M. M. and Chirkova, E. M. (1968). *Toksikologiya novykh promyshöennykh khimicheskikh veshchestv.* **10,** 64.
Gombault, M. (1880). *Archives de Neurologie (Paris)* **1,** 11.
Gonatas, N. K. and Robbins, E. (1965). *Protoplasma* **59,** 377.
Gontzea, J., Dumitrache, S., Rujinski, A. and Cocora, D. (1963). *Internationale Zeitschrift für Angewandte Physilogie, Arbeitsphysiologie* **20,** 20.
Gontzea, J., Sutzesco, P., Cocora, D. and Lungu, D. (1964a). *Archives des Sciences Physiologiques* **18,** 211.
Gontzea, J., Sutescu, P., Stanciu, V. and Lungu, D. (1964b). *Igiena* **13,** 501.
Gordon, C. C. (1968). *East Helena Reports for Director of Air Pollution, 16 December.*
Gordon, N., King, E. and Mackay, R. I. (1967). *British Medical Journal* **2,** 480.
Gould, S. E., Kullman, H. J. and Shecket, H. A. (1937). *American Journal of Medical Science* **194,** 304.
Government Chemist (1968). "1967 Report of the Government Chemist." H.M.S.O., London.
Gowland, W. (1912). *Journal of the Anthropological Institute* **42,** 235.
Goyer, R. A. (1968). *Laboratory Investigation* **19,** 71.
Goyer, R. A. and Krall, R. (1969). *Journal of Cell Biology* **41,** 393.
Goyer, R. A., Krall, R. and Kimball, J. P. (1968). *Laboratory Investigation* **19,** 78.

Goyer, R. A., Leonard, D. L., Moore, J. F., Rhyne, B. and Krigman, M. R. (1970). *Archives of Environmental Health* **20,** 705.
Goyer, R. A. and Mahaffey, K. R. (1972). *Environmental Health Perspectives* No. 2, 73.
Graef, J. W., Kopito, L. and Schwachman, H. (1971). *Postgraduate Medicine,* **50,** 133.
Granati, A., Scavo, D. and Peruzy, A. D. (1956). *Folıa Medica (Napoli)* **39,** 853.
Granick, S. and Mauzerall, D. (1958). *Journal of Biological Chemistry* **232,** 1119.
Grazianni, G., Fusco, M. and Rossi, L. (1954). *Folia Medica (Napoli)* **37,** 643.
Grazianni, G., Pecora, L. and Rossi, L. (1956). *Folia Medica (Napoli)* **39,** 217.
Grazianni, G. and Sessa, T. (1952). *Folia Medica (Napoli)* **35,** 537.
Greenbaum, D., Richardson, P. C., Salmon, M. V. and Urich, H. (1964). *Brain* **87,** 201.
Greenfield, I. and Gray, I. (1950). *American Heart Journal* **39,** 430.
Grigarzik, H. and Passow, H. (1958). *Pflügers Archiv für die Gesamte Physiologie des Menschen und der Tiere* **267,** 73.
Griggs, R. C. (1964). *In* "Progress in Hematology" Vol. 4, p. 117. Grune and Stratton, New York.
Griggs, R. C. and Harris, J. W. (1958). *Clinical Research* **6,** 188.
Griggs, R. C., Sunshine, I., Newill, V. A., Newton, B. W., Buchanan, S. and Rasch, C. A. (1964). *Journal of the American Medical Association* **187,** 703.
Guinee, V. F. (1971). *Transactions of the New York Academy of Science* **33,** 539.
Guinee, V. F. (1972). *American Journal of Medicine* **52,** 283.
Gusev, M. I. (1960). *In* "Maximum Permissible Concentrations of Air Pollutants" (V. A. Ryaznov ed.) Vol. 4, p. 5. Medgiz, Moscow.
Gutniak, P., Koziołowa, H. and Kowalski, E. (1964). *Lancet* **1,** 1137.
Haeger-Aronsen, B. (1960). *Scandinavian Journal of Clinical and Laboratory Investigation* **12,** Suppl. 47.
Haeger-Aronsen, B. (1962). *Scandinavian Journal of Clinical and Laboratory Investigation* **14,** 397.
Haeger-Aronsen, B. (1964). *Pharmacologica et Toxicologica* **21,** 105.
Haeger-Aronsen, B., Abdulla, M. and Fristedt, B. I. (1971). *Archives of Environmental Health* **23,** 440.
Halaceva, L., Boyadziev, V. and Nikolova, P. (1968). *Scripta Scientifica Medica* **6,** 93.
Haley, T. J. (1966). *Archives of Environmental Health* **12,** 781
Hall, A. (1905). *British Medical Journal* **1,** 584.
Hall, A. and Ransom, W. B. (1906). *British Medical Journal* **1,** 428.
Hamilton, A. (1929). "Industrial Poisons in the United States." MacMillan, New York.
Hamilton, A., Reznikoff, P. and Burnham, G. M. (1925). *Journal of the American Medical Association* **84,** 1481.
Hamilton, W. L. and Miller, J. E. (1971). *Ohio Journal of Science* **71,** 313.
Hammer, D. I., Finklea, J. F., Hendricks, R. H., Shy, C. M. and Horton, R. J. M. (1971). *American Journal of Epidemiology* **93,** 84.
Hammond, P. B. (1969). *In* "Essays in Toxicology" (F. R. Blood ed.). Vol. 1, p. 115. Academic Press, New York.
Hammond, P. B. and Aronsen, A. L. (1964). *Annals of the New York Academy of Science* **111,** 595.
Hammond, P. B., Wright, H. N. and Roepke, M. H. (1956). *University of Minnesota Agricultural Experimental Station Technical Bulletin No. 221.*
Hanke, J. Z. (1963). *Medycynya Pracy* **14,** 223.
Hanke, J. Z. (1964). *Archiv za Higijenu Rada i Toksikolgiju* **15,** 57.

Hänninen, H. (1971). *British Journal of Industrial Medicine* **28,** 374.
Hansmann, G. and Perry, M. C. (1940). *Archives of Pathology* **30,** 226.
Hardy, H. L. (1966). *Clinical Pharmacology and Therapeutics* **7,** 713.
Hardy, H. L., Chamberlin, R. I., Maloof, C. C., Boylen, G. W. and Howell, M. C. (1971). *Clinical Pharmacology and Therapeutics* **12,** 982.
Harris, C. E. C. (1958). *Canadian Medical Association Journal* **79,** 664.
Harris, E. B., MacGibbon, B. H. and Mollin, D. L. (1965). *British Journal of Haematology* **11,** 99.
Harris, J. W. and Greenberg, M. S. (1954). *Clinical Research Proceedings* **2,** 55.
Harris, P. W. and Elsea, W. R. (1967). *Journal of the American Medical Association* **202,** 544.
Harris, P. W. and Holley, M. R. (1972). *Pediatrics* **49,** 606.
Harrison, G. E., Carr, T. E. F., Sutton, A. and Humphries, E. R. (1969). *Nature* **224,** 1115.
Harrold, G. C. (1949). *Journal of Industrial Hygiene* **31,** 327.
Hartl, W. and Resch, W. (1972). International Symposium, Environmental Health Aspects of Lead, Amsterdam, Paper 84.
Hasan, J. and Hernberg, S. (1966). *Archives of Environmental Health* **12,** 26.
Hasan, J., Hernberg, S., Metsälä, P., and Vihko, V. (1967a). *Archives of Environmental Health* **14,** 309.
Hasan, J., Vihko, V. and Hernberg, S. (1967b). *Archives of Environmental Health* **14,** 313.
Hass, G. M., Brown, D. V. L., Eisenstein, R. and Hemmens, A. (1964). *American Journal of Pathology* **45,** 691.
Hatch, T. F. and Gross, P. (1964). "Pulmonary Deposition and Retention of Inhaled Aerosols." Academic Press, New York.
Hausman, R., Sturtevant, R. A. and Wilson, W. J. (1961). *J. Forensic Sciences* **6,** 180.
Hausmanowa-Petrusewicz, I., Emeryk, B., Sobkowicz, H., Wasonicz, B. and Tur, J. (1962). *Polski Tygodnik Lekarski* **17,** 1405.
Hay, W. (1950). *British Journal of Industrial Medicine* **7,** 177.
Heller, A. and Kettner, H. (1968). "Probenahme und Bestimung Kleinster Bleimengun in der Luft." VDL-Kommission Reinhaltung der Luft.
Hemphill, F. E., Kaeberle, M. L. and Buck, W. B. (1971). *Science* **172,** 1031.
Henderson, D. A. (1954). *Australian Annals of Medicine* **3,** 219.
Henderson, D. A. (1955). *Australian Annals of Medicine* **4,** 163.
Henderson, D. A. (1958). *Medical Journal of Australia* **1,** 377.
Henderson, D. A. and Inglis, J. A. (1957). *Australian Annals of Medicine* **6,** 145.
Henderson, S. R. and Snyder, L. J. (1961). *Analytical Chemistry* **33,** 1172.
Her Majesty's Factory Inspectorate (1971a). "Methods for the Detection of Toxic Substances in Air. No. 14. Lead and Compounds of Lead." H.M.S.O., London.
Her Majesty's Factory Inspectorate (1971b). "Technical Data No. 16. Prevention of Industrial Lead Poisoning." H.M.S.O., London.
Her Majesty's Factory Inspectorate (1971c). "CMA's Notes of Guidance: Lead." Department of Employment, London.
Her Majesty's Factory Inspectorate (1972). "Threshold Limit Values For 1971." H.M.S.O., London.
Hernberg, S. (1967). *Work—Environment—Health* **3,** Suppl. 1.
Hernberg, S. and Nikkanen, J. (1970). *Lancet* **1,** 63.
Hernberg, S., Lilius, H., Mellin, G. and Nikkanen, J. (1969). *Work—Environment—Health* **6,** 5.
Hernberg, S., Nurminen, M. and Hasan, J. (1967a). *Environmental Research* **1,** 247.

Hernberg, S., Nurminen, M. and Hasan, J. (1967b). *Archiv für Gewerbepathologie und Gewerbehygiene* **23,** 117.
Hernberg, S., Vihko, V. and Hasan, J. (1967c). *Archives of Environmental Health* **14,** 319.
Hernberg, S., Nikkanen, J., Mellin, G. and Lilius, H. (1970). *Archives of Environmental Health* **21,** 140.
Hernberg, S., Tola, S., Nikkanen, J. and Valkonen, S. (1972). *Archives of Environmental Health* **25,** 109.
Herter, C. A. (1895). *New York Medical Journal* **61,** 665.
Hess, J. W. (1961). *New England Journal of Medicine* **264,** 382.
Hettche, H. O. (1964). *International Journal of Air and Water Pollution* **8,** 185.
Hevesy, G. and Nylin, G. (1953). *Circulation Research* **1,** 102.
Hicks, B. B., Nelson, D. M. and Brar, S. S. (1966). *Argonne National Laboratory of Biological Medicine Research Division Annual Report ANL-7278,* p. 307.
Hicks, R. M. (1972). *Chemico-Biological Interactions* **5,** 361.
Hill, C. R. and Jaworowski, Z. S. (1961). *Nature* **190,** 353.
Hirschler, D. A. and Gilbert, L. F. (1964). *Archives of Environmental Health* **8,** 297.
Hirschler, D. A., Gilbert, L. F., Lamb, F. W. and Niebylski, L. M. (1957). *Industrial and Engineering Chemistry* **49,** 1131.
Hofmann, K. B. (1883). *Archiv für Geschichte der Medizin* **6,** 26.
Hofmann, K. B. (1885). "Das Blei bei den Völkern des Alterthums." Hagel, Berlin.
Hofreuter, D. H., Catcott, E. J., Keenan, R. G. and Zintaras, C. (1961). *Archives of Environmental Health* **3,** 568.
Högger, D. (1971). *Bulletin des Eidgenössischen Gesundheitsamtes* **B3.**
Holmqvist, I. (1960). *Schriften. Gesellschaft Deutscher Metallhütten-und Bergleute* **7,** 115.
Holtzman, R. B. (1963). *Health Physics* **9,** 385.
Holtzman, R. B. (1970). *Environmental Science and Technology* **4,** 314.
Honjin, R., Nakamura, R. and Imura, M. (1959). *Okajima Folia Anatomica Japonica* **33,** 131.
Hopkins, A. (1970). *British Journal of Industrial Medicine* **27,** 130.
Horiuchi, K. (1965). *Osaka City Medical Journal* **11,** 225.
Hoschek, R. (1961). *Medizinische Welt.* **2,** 2687.
Howard, J. K. (1972). *Lancet* **2,** 545.
Huff, L. C. (1952). *Economic Geology* **47,** 517.
Humperdinck, K. (1948). *Ärztliche Forschung* **2,** 119.
Hunter, D. (1955). "The Diseases of Occupations." E.U.P. London.
Hunter, D. (1969). "The Diseases of Occupations," 4th Edition. E.U.P. London.
Hunter, D. and Aub, J. C. (1926–1927). *Quarterly Journal of Medicine* **20,** 123.
Hursh, J. B. and Mercer, T. T. (1970). *Journal of Applied Physiology* **28,** 268.
Hursh, J. B. and Suomela, J. (1968). *Acta Radiologica Ther. Physica Biologica* **7,** 108.
Hursh, J. B., Schraub, A., Sattler, E. L. and Hofmann, H. P. (1969). *Health Physics* **16,** 257.
Hutchison, H. E. and Stark, J. M. (1961). *Journal of Clinical Pathology* **14,** 548.
ILO/WHO Committee (1968). "Permissible Levels of Toxic Substances in the Working Environment." International Labour Office, Geneva.
Imamura, Y. (1957). *Osaka City Medical Journal* **3,** 167.
Ingalls, T. H., Tiboni, E. A. and Werrin, M. (1961). *Archives of Environmental Health* **3,** 575.
Institute of Petroleum Atmospheric Committee (1971). *Petroleum Review* **25,** 289.
Ireland, F. E. (1972). "108th Annual Report on Alkali, &c. Works, 1971." H.M.S.O., London.

Jacobi, W. (1964). *Health Physics* **10,** 1163.
Jacobs, J. M., Cavanagh, J. B. and Mellick, R. S. (1966). *British Journal of Experimental Pathology* **47,** 507.
James, L. F., Lazar, V. A. and Binns, W. (1966). *American Journal of Veterinary Research* **27,** 132.
Jandl, J. H. (1960). *Journal of Laboratory and Clinical Medicine* **55,** 663.
Jandl, J. H., Inman, J. K., Simmons, R. L. and Allen, D. W. (1959). *Journal of Clinical Investigation* **38,** 161.
Jarrett, A., Rimington, C. and Willoughby, D. A. (1956). *Lancet* **1,** 125.
Jaulmes, P. (1962). *Montpellier Médical* **61,** 9.
Jaworowski, Z. S. (1963). Thesis, Warsaw.
Jaworowski, Z. S. (1967). *Review Reports of the Nuclear Energy Information Centre, Warsaw,* No. 29.
Jaworowski, Z. S. (1968). *Nature* **217,** 152.
Jecklin, L. (1956). *Archiv für Gewerbepathologie und Gewerbehygiene* **14,** 626.
Jenkins, C. D. and Mellins, R. B. (1957). *Archives of Neurology and Psychiatry* **77,** 70.
Jensen, W. N. and Moreno, G. (1964). *Compte Rendu Hebdomadaire des Séances de l'Académie des Sciences (Paris)* **258,** 3596.
Jensen, W. N., Moreno, G. and Bessis, M. (1965). *Blood* **25,** 933.
Jernigan, E. L., Ray, B. J. and Duce, R. A. (1971). *Atmospheric Environment* **5,** 881.
Johnstone, R. T. (1948). "Occupational Medicine and Industrial Hygiene." Mosby, St. Louis.
Johnstone, R. T. (1966). *Archives of Environmental Health* **12,** 134.
Jonek, J., Kośmider, S. and Grzybek, H. (1963). *Archivum Immunologiæ et Therapiæ Experimentalis* **11,** 652.
Jonek, J., Jonek, T. and Kośmider, S. (1965). *Medycyna Pracy* **16,** 211.
Jones, J. R. E. (1938). *Journal of Experimental Biology* **15,** 394.
Jones, L. H. P. and Clement, C. R. (1972). *In* "Lead in the Environment" (P. Hepple ed.) p. 29. Institute of Petroleum, London.
Jones, R. D., Commins, B. T. and Cernik, A. A. (1972). *Lancet* **2,** 302.
Jost, D., Müller, J. and Jendricke, U. (1972). International Symposium, Environmental Health Aspects of Lead; Amsterdam, Paper 83.
Jowett, M. (1932). *Biochemical Journal* **26,** 2108.
Joyce, C. R. B., Moore, H. A. and Weatherall, M. (1954). *British Journal of Pharmacology* **9,** 463.
Jung, F. (1947). *Archives of Experimental and Pathological Pharmacology* **204,** 139.
Jung, F. (1956). *Folia Haematologica* **73,** 401.
Kahan, V. L. (1950). *Journal of Mental Science* **96,** 1043.
Kammholz, L. P., Thatcher, L. G., Blodgett, F. M. and Good, T. A. (1972). *Pediatrics* **50,** 625.
Kanner, N. L. (1965). *Problemy Endokrinologii i Gormontherapii* **11,** 82.
Kapetonović, K., Radmić, S. and Soldatović, D. (1960). *Acta Pharmaceutica Jugoslavica* **10,** 125.
Karhausen, L. R. (1972). International Symposium, Environmental Health Aspects of Lead, Amsterdam, Paper 39.
Karlog, O. and Møller, K. O. (1958). *Acta Pharmacologica et Toxicologica* **15,** 8.
Karnofsky, D. A. and Ridgway, L. P. (1952). *Journal of Pharmacology and Experimental Therapeutics* **104,** 176.
Karpatkin, S. (1961). *Archives of Environmental Health* **2,** 679.
Kaye, S. and Reznikoff, P. (1947). *Journal of Industrial Hygiene* **29,** 178.

Kehoe, R. A. (1925). *Journal of the American Medical Association* **85,** 108.
Kehoe, R. A. (1927). *Journal of Laboratory and Clinical Medicine* **12,** 554.
Kehoe, R. A. (1961a). *Journal of the Royal Institute of Public Health* **24,** 101; 129; 177; 203.
Kehoe, R. A. (1961b). *Pure and Applied Chemistry* **3,** 129.
Kehoe, R. A. (1964a). *Archives of Environmental Health* **8,** 235.
Kehoe, R. A. (1964b). *Lancet* **2,** 594.
Kehoe, R. A. (1968). *Science* **189,** 1000.
Kehoe, R. A. (1969). *Atmospheric Environment* **3,** 87.
Kehoe, R. A. (1972). *Journal of Occupational Medicine* **14,** 390.
Kehoe, R. A. and Thamann, F. (1931). *American Journal of Hygiene* **13,** 478.
Kehoe, R. A., Thamann, F. and Cholak, J. (1933a). *Journal of Industrial Hygiene* **15,** 257.
Kehoe, R. A., Thamann, F. and Cholak, J (1933b). *Journal of Industrial Hygiene* **15,** 273.
Kehoe, R. A. and Thamann, F. (1933c). *Journal of Industrial Hygiene* **15,** 290
Kehoe, R. A., Thamann, F. and Cholak, J. (1933d). *Journal of Industrial Hygiene* **15,** 301.
Kehoe, R. A., Thamann, F. and Cholak, J. (1934). *Journal of Industrial Hygiene* **16,** 100.
Kehoe, R. A., Thamann, F. and Cholak, J. (1936). *Journal of Industrial Hygiene* **18,** 42.
Kehoe, R. A., Cholak, J., Hubbard, D. M., Bambach, K., McNary, R. R. and Strong, R. V. (1940a). *Journal of Industrial Hygiene* **22,** 381.
Kehoe, R. A., Cholak, J. and Story, R. V. (1940b). *Journal of Nutrition* **19,** 579.
Kehoe, R. A., Cholak, J., Hubbard, D. M., Bambach, K. and McNary, R. R. (1943). *Journal of Industrial Hygiene* **25,** 71.
Kehoe, R. A., Cholak, J. and Spence, J. A. (1963). *Archives of Environmental Health* **6,** 239.
Keppler, J. F., Maxfield, M. E. and Moss, W. D. (1970). *American Industrial Hygiene Association Journal* **31,** 412.
Kifune, I., Sugai, R., Urishiyama, Y. and Abe, E. (1970). *Nigata Prefecture Public Health Laboratory Meetings Abstracts* **21-22.**
Kilham, L., Low, R. J., Conti, S. F. and Dallenbach, D. C. (1962). *Journal of the National Cancer Institute* **29,** 863.
King, B. G. (1971). *American Journal of Diseases of Children* **122,** 337.
King, E. and Thompson, A. R. (1961). *Annals of Occupational Hygiene* **3,** 247.
Kiryakov, K. (1959). *Süvremenna Meditsina* **10,** 42.
Kiryakov, S. (1963). *Proceedings of the Bulgarian Society of Neurology and Psychiatry. Section of EGG and Clinical Neurophysiology, Sofia,* p. 709.
Klein, J. R. (1962). *American Journal of Physiology* **203,** 971.
Klein, M., Namer, R., Harpur, E. and Corbin, R. (1970). *New England Journal of Medicine* **283,** 669.
Kline, T. S. (1960). *American Journal of Diseases of Children* **99,** 48.
Kloke, A., Reibartsch, K. and Leh, H. (1966). *Zeitschrift für Landwissenschaftliches Versuchs und Untersuchungswesen* **20,** 119.
Knelson, J. H., Johnson, R. J., Coulston, F., Goldberg, L. and Griffin, T. (1972). International Symposium, Environmental Health Aspects of Lead, Amsterdam, Paper 36.
Kobayashi, J. (1957). *Bericht des Ōhara Instituts* **11,** 12.
Kolkovski, P. and Rajceva, V. (1961). *Archiv für Toxikologie* **19,** 237.
Kopito, L., Byers, R. K. and Schwachman, H. (1967). *New England Journal of Medicine* **276,** 949.
Kośmider, S. (1953). *Archiv für Gewerbepathologie und Gewerbehygiene* **20,** 11.
Kośmider, S. (1963). *Polskie Archiwum Medycyny Wewnetrznej* **32,** 1253.

Kośmider, S. and Petelenz, T. (1962). *Polskie Archiwum Medycyny Wewnetrznej* **32,** 437.

Kośmider, S. and Petocka, Z. (1967). *Zentralblatt für Arbeitsmedizin und Arbeitsschutz* **17,** 170.

Kośmider, S. and Sroczyński, J. (1961). *Postepy Higieny i Medycyny Doswiadozalnej* **15,** 353.

Kostial, K., Duraković, A., Šimonović, I. and Juvančić, V. (1969). *International Journal of Radiation Biology* **15,** 563.

Kostial, K., Šimonović, I. and Pišonić, M. (1971a). Communication at 3rd Yugoslav Congress of Industrial Medicine, Lijubljana.

Kostial, K., Šimonović, I. and Pišonić, M. (1971b). *Nature* **233,** 564.

Kostial, K., Šimonović, I and Pišonić, M. (1971c). *Environmental Research* **4,** 360.

Kostial, K. and Vouk, V. B. (1957). *British Journal of Pharmacology* **12,** 219.

Kotok, D. (1972). *Journal of Pediatrics* **80,** 57.

Kradel, D. C., Adams, W. M. and Guss, S. B. (1965). *Veterinary Medicine* **60,** 1045.

Kraut, H. and Weber, M. (1944). *Biochemische Zeitschrift* **317,** 133.

Kreiner-Birnbaum, M. and Grinstein, M. (1965). *Biochemica Biophysica Acta* **108,** 110.

Kremer, H. V. and Martin, F. N. (1955). *Annals of Internal Medicine* **42,** 1130.

de Kretser, A. J. and Waldron, H. A, (1963a). *British Journal of Industrial Medicine* **20,** 35

de Kretser, A. J. and Waldron, H. A. (1963b). *British Journal of Industrial Medicine* **20,** 316.

de Kretser, A. J. and Waldron, H. A. (1965). *British Journal of Industrial Medicine* **22,** 315.

Krigman, M. R., Crane, D. and Goyer, R. A. (1968). *Federation of American Societies for Experimental Biology* **27,** 40.

Krücke, W. (1941). *Virchows Archiv für Pathologische Anatomie und Physiologie und für Klinische Medizin* **308,** 1.

Kubota, J., Lazar, V. A. and Losee, F. (1968). *Archives of Environmental Health* **16,** 788.

Kumashiro, K. and Ogata, M. (1971). *Igaku to Seibutsugaku,* **82,** 89.

Lahmann, E. and Möller, M. (1967). *Bundesges.* **17,** 261.

Lampert, P. W. and Schochet, S. S. (1968). *Journal of Neuropathology and Experimental Neurology* **27,** 401.

Lampert, P. W., Garrow, G. and Pentschew, A. (1967). *In* "Brain Edema" (I Klatzo and F. Seitelberger eds.) p. 207. Springer Verlag, New York.

Lancéreaux, E. (1881a). *Archives Générales de Médecine* **6,** 641.

Lancéreaux, E. (1881b). *Transactions of the International Medical Congress* Vol. 2, p. 193.

Lancet (1973). **1,** 87.

Landing, B. H. and Nakai, H. (1959). *American Journal of Clinical Pathology* **31,** 499.

Lane, R. E. (1949). *British Journal of Industrial Medicine* **6,** 125.

Lane, R. E. (1964). *Archives of Environmental Health* **8,** 243.

Lane, R. E. and Lewy, F. H. (1935). *Journal of Industrial Hygiene* **17,** 79.

Lane, R. E., Hunter, D., Malcolm, D., Williams, M. K., Hudson, T. G. F., Browne, R. C., McCallum, R. I., Thompson, A. R., de Kretser, A. J., Zielhuis, R. L., Cramér, K., Barry, P. S. I., Goldberg, A., Beritić, T., Vigliani, E. C., Truhaut, R., Kehoe, R. A. and King, E. (1968). *British Medical Journal* **4,** 501.

Lang, E. P. and Kunze, F. M. (1948). *Journal of Industrial Hygiene* **30,** 256.

de Langen, C. D. and ten Berg, J. A. G. (1948). *Acta Medica Scandinavica* **130,** 37.

Lanzola, E., Allegrini, M. and Breuer, F. (1972). International Symposium, Environmental Health Aspects of Lead, Amsterdam, Paper 31.

Larizza, P. and Ventura, S. (1954). *Medicina (Parma)* **4,** 1.

Larsen, A. A. (1969). Report of Inter-Agency Committee on Environmental Study.
Laslett, E. E. and Warrington, W. B. (1898). *Brain* **21,** 224.
Laveskog, A. (1971). *In* "Proceedings of the Second Clean Air Congress" (H. M. England and W. T. Beery eds.) p. 549. Academic Press, New York.
Law, W. R. and Nelson, E. R. (1968). *Journal of the American Medical Association* **204,** 1002.
Lawther, P. J., Commins, B. T., Ellison, J. McK. and Biles, B. (1972). *In* "Lead in the Environment" (P. Hepple ed.) p. 8. Institute of Petroleum, London.
Lazrus, A. L., Lorange, E. and Lodge, J. P. (1970). *Environmental Science and Technology* **4,** 55.
Lebbe, M. J. (1965). *Pollution Atmosphérique* **7,** 316.
Lederer, L. B. and Bing, F. G. (1940). *Journal of the American Medical Association* **114,** 2457.
Lee, R. E., Patterson, R. K. and Wagman, J. (1968). *Environmental Science and Technology* **2,** 288.
Legge, T. M. and Goadby, K. W. (1912). "Lead Poisoning and Lead Absorption." Arnold, London.
Lehmann, L. and Sittkus, A. (1959). *Naturwissenschaften* **46,** 9.
Lehnert, G. (1969). *Archiv für Hygiene und Bakteriologie* **152,** 559.
Leikin, S. and Eng, G. (1963). *Pediatrics* **31,** 996.
Leone, A. J. (1968). *American Journal of Roentgenology* **103,** 165.
Levinson, A. and Zeldes, M. (1939). *Archives of Pediatrics* **56,** 738.
Lewis, K. H. (1966). "Symposium on Environmental Lead Contamination." U.S. Public Health Service Publication No. 1440, p. 17.
Leyden, E. (1883). *Deutsche Medizinische Wochenschrift* **19,** 185.
Lichtman, H. C. and Feldman, F. (1963). *Journal of Clinical Investigation* **42,** 830.
Linari, F., Coscia, G. C., Martorano, G. and Perrelli, G. (1963). *Archives des Sciences Médicales* **116,** 336.
Lind, G. (1936). *Journal of Industrial Hygiene* **18,** 37.
Lindemann, R. and Assenzo, J. (1964). *American Journal of Public Health* **54,** 1071.
Lin-Fu, J. S. (1967). U.S. Department of Health, Education and Welfare, Social and Rehabilitation Service, Children's Bureau Publication 452, U.S. Government Printing Office, Washington.
Lin-Fu, J. S. (1972). *New England Journal of Medicine* **286,** 702.
Liniger, R. L., Duce, R. A., Winchester, J. W. and Matson, W. R. (1966). *Journal of Geophysical Research* **71,** 2457.
Livesley, B. and Sissons, C. E. (1968). *British Medical Journal* **4,** 387.
Lloyd-Davies, T. A. (1972). "Annual Report of H.M. Inspector of Factories, 1971." H.M.S.O., London.
Lob, M. and Desbaumes, P. (1971). *Schweizerische Medizinische Wochenschrift* **101,** 357.
Locke, L. N., Bagley, G. E. and Irby, H. D. (1966). *Bulletin, Wildlife Disease Association* **2,** 127.
Locke, L. N., Bagley, G. E. and Young, L. T. (1967). *Bulletin, Wildlife Disease Association* **3,** 176.
Loewe, O. (1906). *Archives of Ophthalmology* **35,** 164.
Lothe, K. and Falbe-Hansen, I. (1963). *Clinical Science* **24,** 47.
Lovelock, J. E. (1955). *Biochemical Journal* **60,** 692.
Ludwig, G. D. (1957). *Archives of Internal Medicine* **100,** 802.
Lundgren, D. A. (1970). *Journal of the Air Pollution Control Association* **20,** 603.
MacFadzean, A. J. S. and Davis, L. J. (1947). *Glasgow Medical Journal* **28,** 537.

MacFadzean, A. J. S. and Davis, L. J. (1949). *Quarterly Journal of Medicine* **18,** 57.
McCann, F. B. (1932). *In* "Interim Report of an Official Enquiry into the Chronic Nephritis of Queensland With Special Reference to Plumbism in Children." (R. W. Cilento ed.) Department of Health, Commonwealth of Australia, Brisbane, p. 66.
McClain, R. M. and Becker, B. A. (1972). *Toxicology and Applied Pharmacology* **21,** 265.
McCord, C. (1953). *Industrial Medicine* **22,** 573.
McDonald, N. S., Erzimilian, F., Spain, P. and McArthur, C. (1951). *Journal of Biological Chemistry* **189,** 387.
McGillion, F. and Goldberg, A. (1973). (In press.)
McIntyre, M. S. and Angle, C. R. (1972). *Science* **177,** 520.
McKhann, C. F. (1932). *Archives of Neurology and Psychiatry, Chicago* **27,** 294.
McKhann, C. F. and Vogt, E. C. (1933). *Journal of the American Medical Association* **101,** 1131.
McLaughlin, J., Marliac, J.-P., Verrett, M. J., Mutchler, M. K. and Fitzhugh, O. G. (1963). *Toxicology and Applied Pharmacology* **6,** 760.
McLaughlin, M. C. (1956). *New York State Journal of Medicine* **56,** 3711.
McLean, R., Calhoun, J. A. and Aub, J. C. (1954). *Archives of Industrial Health* **9,** 113.
McRoberts, W. J. (1973). *Journal of the Society of Occupational Medicine* **23,** 3.
Machle, W. F. (1935). *Journal of the American Medical Association* **105,** 378.
Magistretti, M., Pierone, E. and Majoni, A. (1961). *Medicina del Lavoro* **52,** 498.
Makashev, M. K. and Verbolovich, V. P. (1967). *Izvestia Akademii Nauk SSSR Series Biol* **5,** 59.
Malcolm, D. (1971). *Archives of Environmental Health* **23,** 292.
Maloof, C. C. (1950). *Archives of Industrial Hygiene* **1,** 296.
Manley, C. H. (1937). *Analyst* **62,** 544.
Mann, T. S. (1962). *Scottish Medical Journal* **7,** 36.
Marie, P. and Bertrand, I. (1918). *Annales Médicales* **5,** 209.
Marsden, H. B. and Wilson, V. K. (1955). *British Medical Journal* **1,** 324.
Maseroni, R. (1969). *Bulletin of the World Health Organization* **40,** 305.
Massione, R. (1941). *Medicina del Lavoro* **32,** 149.
Massurovsky, E. B., Bunge, M. B. and Bunge, R. P. (1967). *Journal of Cell Biology* **32,** 497.
Maxwell, L. C. and Bischoff, F. (1929a). *Journal of Pharmacological and Experimental Theraeutics* **36,** 279.
Maxwell, L. C. and Bischoff, F. (1929b). *Journal of Pharmacological and Experimental Therapeutics* **37,** 413.
Mayers, H. R. (1947). *Occupational Medicine* **3,** 77.
Mayers, M. R. (1927). *Journal of Industrial Hygiene* **9,** 239.
Mehani, S. (1966). *Annals of Occupational Hygiene* **9,** 165.
Mellins, R. B. and Jenkins, C. D. (1955). *Journal of the American Medical Association* **158,** 15.
Meo, G., Martorano, G., Bonzanino, A. and Perrelli, G. (1964). *Bollettino della Società Italiana di Biologia Sperimentale* **40,** 649.
Mertz, W., Roginski, E. E. and Schwartz, K. (1961). *Journal of Biological Chemistry* **236,** 318.
Mertz, W., Roginski, E. E. and Schroeder, H. A. (1965). *Journal of Nutrition* **86,** 107.
Milic, S., Stankovic, M., Delic, V. and Djordjevic, V. (1972). International Symposium, Environmental Health Aspects of Lead, Amsterdam, Paper 53.
Millar, J. A., Battistini, V., Cumming, R. I. C., Carswell, F. and Goldberg, A. (1970). *Lancet* **2,** 695.

Millar, J. A., Thompson, G. G., Goldberg, A., Barry, P. S. I. and Lowe, E. H. (1972). *British Journal of Industrial Medicine* **29,** 317.
Mills, A. L. (1971). *Chemistry in Britain* **7,** 160.
Minden, H., Zegarski, W. and Rothe, R. (1964). *Archiv für Gewerbepathologie und Gewerbehygiene* **20,** 461.
Minerals Year Book (1970). Vol. 1, United States Department of the Interior, Washington.
Ministry of Agriculture, Fisheries and Food (1972). "Working Party on the Monitoring of Foodstuffs for Heavy Metals. Second Report: Survey of Lead in Food." H.M.S.O., London.
Mitchell, R. L. and Reith, J. S. (1966). *Journal of the Science of Food and Agriculture* **17,** 437.
Molyneux, M. K. B. (1964). *British Journal of Industrial Medicine* **21,** 203.
Moncrieff, A. A., Koumides, O. P., Clayton, B. E., Patrick, A. D., Renwick, G. C. and Roberts, G. E. (1964). *Archives of Disease in Childhood* **39,** 1.
Moncrieff, A. A., Clayton, B. E. and Roberts, C. E. (1967). *British Medical Journal* **3,** 174.
Monier-Williams, G. W. (1938). "Lead in Food. Ministry of Health Report No. 88 on Public Health and Medical Subjects." H.M.S.O., London.
Moore, M. R. (1973). *Nature* **243,** 222.
Moosa, A. and Harris, E. (1969). *Clinica Pediatrica* **8,** 400.
Morgan, E. H. and Laurell, C.-B. (1963). *British Journal of Haematology* **9,** 471.
Morgan, J. M. (1972). *Archives of Environmental Health* **25,** 26.
Morgan, J. M., Hartley, M. W. and Miller, R. E. (1966). *Archives of Internal Medicine* **118,** 17.
Morris, C. E., Heyman, A. and Pozefsky, T. (1964). *Neurology* **14,** 493.
Morris, H. P. (1940). *Journal of Industrial Hygiene* **22,** 100.
Morris, J. N., Crawford, M. D. and Heady, J. A. (1961). *Lancet* **1,** 860.
Morris, J. N., Crawford, M. D. and Heady, J. A. (1962). *Lancet* **2,** 506.
Morrow, J. J., Urata, G. and Goldberg, A. (1969). *Clinical Science* **37,** 533.
Mortensen, R. A. (1942). *Journal of Industrial Hygiene* **24,** 285.
Mortensen, R. A. and Kellogg, K. E. (1944). *Journal of Cellular and Comparative Physiology* **23,** 11.
Mosny, F. and Malloizel, L. (1907). *Revue Médicale, Paris* **27,** 505.
Motto, H. L., Daines, R. H., Chilko, D. M. and Motto, C. K. (1970). *Environmental Science and Technology* **4,** 231.
Moyers, J. L., Zoller, W. H., Duce, R. A. and Hoffman, G. L. (1972). *Environmental Science and Technology* **6,** 68.
Mueller, P. K. and Stanley, R. L. (1970). AIHL Report No. 87. State of California Department of Public Health, Air and Industrial Hygiene Laboratory.
Mueller, P. K., Helwig, H. L., Alcocer, A. E., Gong, W. K. and Jones, E. E. (1963). *American Society for Testing Materials Standards and Tentative Standards, Special Technical Publication* **352,** 60.
Mulcahahy, R. (1964). *Journal of the Irish Medical Association* **55,** 17.
Mulcahahy, R. (1966). *British Medical Journal* **1,** 861.
Mulcahahy, R. (1968). *Lancet* **1,** 975.
Müller, H. A. and Stöcker, E. (1964). *Experientia* **20,** 379.
Müller, J. (1950). *Praktyka Lekarska* **2,** 49.
Muller, M., Fontaine, E. and Leleu, G. (1962). *Archives des Maladies Professionelles de Médecine du Travail et de Sécurité Sociale* **23,** 541.

Munro, D. A. and Solman, V. E. F. (1967). *In* "Canadian Council of Resource Ministers: Background Papers Prepared for National Conference on 'Pollution and Our Environment', October 1966" Vol. 1, p. 1. Montreal.

Muro, L. A. and Goyer, R. A. (1969). *Archives of Pathology* **87**, 660.

Murozumi, M., Chow, T. J. and Patterson, C. C. (1969). *Geochimica Cosmochimica Acta* **33**, 1247.

Murray, R. E. (1939). "Plumbism and Chronic Nephritis in Young People in Queensland." Commonwealth of Australia, Department of Health Service Publication.

Muss, D. L. (1962). *Journal of the American Water Works Association* **54**, 1371.

Myers, P. S. (1971). *Journal of the Washington Academy of Science* **61**, 58.

Myerson, R. M. and Eisenhauer, J. H. (1963). *American Journal of Cardiology* **11**, 409.

Nago, Y. (1959). *Journal of the Osaka City Medical Center* **8**, 499.

Nakamura, T., Namba, T. and Grob, D. (1967). *Journal of Histochemistry and Cytochemistry* **15**, 275.

Nakao, K., Wada, O. and Yano, Y. (1968). *Clinica Chimica Acta* **19**, 319.

Namba, M., Fujita, H., Hijiya, T., Mii, H. and Kobayashi, S. (1961). *Psychiatria et Neurologia Japonica* **63**, 37.

National Research Council, National Academy of Sciences (1971). "Airborne Lead in Perspective." N.A.S., Washington.

Needleman, H. C., Tuncay, O. C. and Shapiro, I. M. (1972). *Nature* **235**, 111.

Nelson, J. D., Dorn, P., Rogers, L. E. and Sartain, P. (1968). *American Journal of Clinical Pathology* **50**, 297.

Newton-John, H. F. and Morgan, D. B. (1968). *Lancet* **1**, 232.

Nieburg, P. (1972). *Journal of Pediatrics* **80**, 627.

Nishiyama, S. (1957). *Shikoku Acta Medica* **11**, 164.

Norris, C. and Gettler, A. O. (1925). *Journal of the American Medical Association* **85**, 818.

Nunziante-Cesaro, A., Granata, A. and Saita, G. (1956). *Folia Medica (Napoli)* **39**, 132.

Nusbaum, R. E., Butt, E. M., Golmour, T. C. and DiDio, S. L. (1965). *Archives of Environmental Health* **10**, 227.

Nye, L. J. J. (1929). *Medical Journal of Australia* **2**, 145.

Nye, L. J. J. (1933). "Chronic Nephritis and Lead Poisoning." Angus and Robertson, Sydney.

Oliver, T. (1891a). "Lead Poisoning." Bentland, Edinburgh.

Oliver, T. (1891b). *Lancet* **1**, 644.

Oliver, T. (1902). *In* "Dangerous Trades" (T. Oliver ed.) p. 282. Murray, London.

Oliver, T. (1911). *British Medical Journal* **1**, 1096.

Oliver, T. (1914). "Lead Poisoning." Lewis, London.

Olliver, A. (1862). *Archives Générales de Médecine* **2**, 530.

Ophlüs, W. (1915). *American Journal of Medical Science* **150**, 518.

Oser, B. L. (1970). *Food and Cosmetics Toxicology* **9**, 245.

Otrzonsek, N. (1967). *Archiv für Gewerbepathologie und Gewerbehygiene* **24**, 66.

Ottoboni, F. and Kahn, E. (1970). Interim Report, California Department of Public Health.

Packham, R. F. (1971). *Water Treatment and Examination* **20**, 144.

Pakhotina, N. S. (1958). *Gigiena i Sanitariya* **23**, 3.

Palmisano, P. A., Sneed, R. C. and Cassady, G. (1969). *Journal of Pediatrics* **75**, 869.

Paolino, W., Resegotti, L., Sartoris, S. and Infelise, V. (1963). *Minerva Medicina* **54**, 527.

Paparopoli, G. (1955). *Bolletino della Società Italiana Biologia Sperimentale* **31**, 1426.

Park, E. A., Jackson, D., Goodwin, T. C. and Kajdi, L. (1933). *Journal of Pediatrics* **3**, 265.

Parnese, E. (1963). *Zeitschrifte für Zellforschung und Mikroskopische Anatomie* **60,** 711.
Parry, W. H. (1967). *Lancet* **2,** 1208.
Partington, J. R. (1935). "Origins and Development of Applied Chemistry." Longmans, London.
Passow, H. and Tillman, K. (1956). *Pflügers Archiv für die Gesamte Physiologie* **262,** 23.
Passow, H., Rothstein, A. and Clarkson, T. W. (1961). *Pharmacological Reviews* **13,** 185.
Patterson, C. C. (1965). *Archives of Environmental Health* **11,** 344.
Patterson, C. C. (1971). *Connecticut Medicine* **35,** 347.
Paul, C. (1860). *Archives Générales de Médecine* **15,** 513.
Pecora, L., Pesarsi, C. and Lamanna, A. (1964). *Folia Medica (Napoli)* **47,** 985.
Pejic, S. (1928). *Annals of Internal Medicine* **1,** 577.
Pentschew, A. and Garro, F. (1966). *Acta Neuropathologica* **6,** 266.
Perlstein, M. A. and Attala, R. (1966). *Clinical Pediatrics* **5,** 292.
Pernis, B. and Bairati, A. (1959). *Medicina del Lavoro* **50,** 447.
Pernis, B., Bairati, A. and Giubileo, M. (1959). *Medicina del Lavoro* **50,** 107.
Pernis, B. and Finulli, M. (1960). *Medicina del Lavoro* **51,** 481.
Pernis, P., Vigliani, E. L., Depretis, S., Beard, R. and Karlbad, G. (1964). *Proceedings 14th International Congress on Occupational Health, Madrid,* Vol. 2, p. 798.
Perocchia, C. (1966). *Laboratory Investigation* **15,** 479.
Peters, R. A., Stocken, L. A. and Thompson, R. H. S. (1945). *Nature* **156,** 616.
Peterson, E. R. and Murray, M. R. (1960). *Developmental Biology* **2,** 461.
Petrilli, F. L., Agnese, G. and Kanitz, S. (1966). *Archives of Environmental Health* **12,** 733.
Pettinati, L., Rasetti, L. and Rubino, G. (1959). *Rassegna di Medicina Industriale e di Igiena del Lavoro* **28,** 379.
Phelan, P. D. (1959). Thesis, Queensland.
Phillippe, M. and Gothard, M. (1903). *Revue Neurologique* **11,** 117.
Pierrard, J. M. (1969). *Environmental Science and Technology* **3,** 48.
Pinto, S. S., Einert, C., Roberts, W. J., Winn, G. S. and Nelson, K. W. (1952). *Archives of Industrial Hygiene* **6,** 496.
Pinto, S. S., Elkins, H. B. and Ege, J. F. (1941). *Journal of Industrial Hygiene* **23,** 313.
Pisani, W., Bonzanino, A. and Lacquanti, A. (1967). *Medicina del Lavoro* **58,** 279.
Plamieniak, Z. and Smolik, R. (1963). *Polski Tygodrik Lekarski* **18,** 358.
Pomerantseva, E. N. (1950). *Klinische Medizin (Moscow).* **28,** 67.
Popoff, N., Weinberg, S. and Geigin, I. (1963). *Neurology* **13,** 101.
Porritt, N. (1931). *British Medical Journal* **2,** 92.
Posner, A. S. (1969). *Physiological Reviews* **49,** 760.
Powell, K. R. and Rolfe, U. T. (1972). *Journal of Pediatrics* **80,** 628.
Power, J. G. C., Barnes, R. M., Nash, W. N. C. and Robinson, J. B. (1969). *British Medical Journal* **3,** 336.
Prader, A. (1948). *Schweizerische Medizinische Wochenschrift* **78,** 273.
Preiskel, D. (1958). *Annals of Physical Medicine* **4,** 293.
Prendergast, W. D. (1910). *British Medical Journal* **1,** 1164.
Přerovská, I. and Teisinger, J. (1970). *British Journal of Industrial Medicine* **27,** 352.
Prevost, G. L. and Binet, P. (1927). *Revue Medicale de la Suisse Romande* **17,** 444.
Price-Jones, C. (1924–1925). *Medical Science Abstracts and Reviews* **11,** 147.
Prince, A. L. (1957). *Soil Science* **84,** 413.
Pringle, B. H., Hissong, D. E., Katz, E. L. and Mulawka, S. T. (1968). *Proceedings of the American Society of Civil Engineers* **94,** 455.
Prpic-Majic, D., Fugas, M. and Susnik, J. (1972). International Symposium, Environmental Health Aspects of Lead, Amsterdam, Paper 65.

Pueschel, S. M., Kopito, L. and Schwachman, H. (1972). *Journal of the American Medical Association* **222,** 462.

Rabinowitz, M. B. and Wetherill, G. W. (1972). *Environmental Science and Technology* **6,** 705.

Radošević, Z., Šarić, M., Beritić, T. and Knežević, J. (1961). *British Journal of Industrial Medicine* **18,** 222.

Radulescu, I. C., Dinischiotu, G. T., Maugsch, C., Ionescu, C. and Teoderescu-Exarcu, I. (1957). *Archives des Maladies Professionelles de Médecine du Travail et de Sécurité Sociale* **18,** 125.

Rainsford, S. G. (1968). *Proceedings of the Royal Navy Medical Service* **54,** 69.

Rajegowda, B. K., Glass, L. and Evans, H. C. (1972). *Journal of Pediatrics,* **80,** 116.

Rakkimova, M. T. (1968). *Gigiena Truda i Professional' nÿe Zabolevaniya* **12,** 39.

Rameau, J. Th. L. B. (1968). *T.N.O.-Nieuws* **23,** 54.

Rameau, J. Th. L. B. (1972). International Symposium, Environmental Health Aspects of Lead, Amsterdam, Paper 15.

Rapoport, M. and Rubin, M. I. (1941). *American Journal of Disease of Children* **61,** 245.

Rasetti, L. and Parigi, A. (1962). *Folia Medica (Napoli)* **45,** 480.

Rasetti, L., Pettinati, L. and Scansetti, G. (1961). *Proceedings of the 13th International Congress on Occupational Health, New York,* p. 348.

Read, J. L. and Williams, J. P. (1952). *American Heart Journal* **44,** 797.

Reddi, K. K. (1953). *Nature* **172,** 202.

Reed, C. D. and Tolley, J. A. (1967a). *Lancet* **1,** 894.

Reed, C. D. and Tolley, J. A. (1967b). *Lancet* **1,** 1382.

Reed, C. D. and Tolley, J. A. (1967c). *Lancet* **2,** 1258.

Reiders, F. and Brieger, H. (1955). *Proceedings of the 7th Annual Meeting of the American Academy of Occupational Medicine Pa.,* p. 83.

Renshaw, G. D., Pounds, C. A. and Pearson, E. F. (1972). *Nature* **238,** 162.

Richet, G., Albahary, C., Ardaillou, K., Sultan, C. and Morel-Maroger, L. (1964). *Revue Française de Biologie Clinique* **9,** 188.

Richter, G. W., Kress, Y. and Cornwall, C. C. (1968). *American Journal of Pathology* **53,** 189.

Richter, R. H. H. and Schlatter, C. (1971). *Bulletin des Eidgenössischen Gesundheitsamtes Amt. Beil B. Nr. 3.*

Rickword-Lane, C. and Lawrence, A. (1961). *British Medical Journal* **2,** 939.

Rimington, C. (1937). *Compte Rendu des Travaux du Laboratoire de Carlsberg, ser. chim.* **22,** 454.

Rimington, C. (1956). *British Medical Journal* **2,** 189.

Rjazanov, V. A. (1965). *Bulletin of the World Health Organization* **32,** 389.

Robinson, E. and Ludwig, F. (1964). Final Report PA-4788, Stanford Research Institute.

Robinson, M. J., Karminski, F. E. and Brieger, H. (1958). *Pediatrics* **21,** 693.

Rondia, D. and De Graeve, J. (1972). International Symposium, Environmental Health Aspects of Lead, Amsterdam, Paper 89.

Rossi, L. (1955). *Folia Medica (Napoli)* **38,** 1099.

Rossi, L. (1956). *Riforma Medica* **30,** 841.

Rowland, R. E. (1966). *Clinical Orthopedics* **49,** 233.

Rozenberg, P. A. and Smirnova, M. I. (1961). *Gigiena Truda i Professional' nÿe Zabolevaniya* **5,** 35.

Rubino, G. F. (1961). *Panminerva Medica* **3,** 41.

Rubino, G. F. (1962). *Panminerva Medica* **4,** 340.

Rubino, G. F., Prato, V. and Fiorino, L. (1956). *Folia Medica (Napoli)* **39,** 1117.
Rubino, G. F., Pagliardi, E., Prato, V. and Giangrandi, E. (1958). *British Journal of Haematology* **4,** 103.
Rubino, G. F., Prato, V. and Fiorino, L. (1959). *Folia Medica (Napoli)* **42,** 1.
Rubino, G. F., Rasetti, L. and Teso, G. A. (1960). *Proceedings of the 13th International Congress on Occupational Health, New York*, p. 359.
Ruddock, J. C. (1924). *Journal of the American Medical Association* **82,** 1682.
Rühling, A. and Tyler, G. (1968). *Botaniska Notiser* **121,** 321.
Rüssel, H. and Schöberl, A. (1970). *Deutsche Tierärztliche Wochenschrift* **77,** 517.
Russell, R. D. and Farquhar, R. M. (1960). "Lead Isotopes in Geology." Interscience, New York.
Rustagi, J. S. (1964). *Archives of Environmental Health* **8,** 68.
Rustagi, J. S. (1965). *Archives of Environmental Health* **10,** 761.
Ruždig, I. (1950). *Archiv za Higijenu Rada i Toksikolgiju* **1,** 160.
Ryder, H., Cholak, J. and Kehoe, R. A. (1947). *Science* **106,** 63.
Sachs, H. K., Blanksma, L. A., Murray, E. F. and O'Connell, M. J. (1970). *Pediatrics* **46,** 389.
Saita, G. (1959). *Medicina del Lavoro* **50,** 660.
Saita, G. (1960). *Medicina del Lavoro* **51,** 694.
Saita, G. and Moreo, L. (1967). *Medicina del Lavoro* **58,** 364.
Saita, G., Fiocchi, F. and Cattaneo, E. (1952). *Medicina del Lavoro* **43,** 99.
Saita, G., Moreo, L. and Petrocchi, V. (1955). *Medicina del Lavoro* **46,** 463.
Sanders, L. W. (1964). *Archives of Environmental Health* **8,** 270.
Sanders, S. M. (1960). *Health Physics* **2,** 295.
Sandstead, H. H. and Galloway, R. (1967). *Proceedings of the Society for Experimental Biology and Medicine* **124,** 18.
Sandstead, H. H., Brill, A. B., Arias, L., Terry, R. T. and Tinnell, L. E. (1966). *Federation Proceedings. Federation of American Societies for Experimental Biology* **25,** 688.
Sandstead, H. H., Michelakis, A. M. and Temple, T. E. (1970). *Archives of Environmental Health* **20,** 356.
Sano, S. (1958). *Acta Haematologica Japonica* **21,** Suppl. 2.
Sano, S., Inoue, S., Tanabe, Y. and Koike, S. (1959). *Science* **129,** 275.
Sano, S., Inoue, S., Harada, A. and Orita, Z. (1960). *Acta Scholae Medicinalis Universitatis in Kioto* **36,** 182.
Sauer, R. M., Zook, B. C. and Garner, F. M. (1970). *Science* **169,** 1091.
Sautter, A. C. (1922). *American Journal of Ophthalmology* **5,** 468.
Sávay, G. and Csillik, B. (1958). *Nature* **181,** 1137.
Sávay, G. and Csillik, B. (1959). *Experientia* **15,** 396.
Scanlon, J. (1971). *American Journal of Diseases of Childhood* **12,** 325.
Schlaepfer, W. W. (1968). *Journal of Neuropathology and Experimental Neurology* **28,** 401.
Schlaepfer, W. W. and Hager, H. (1964). *American Journal of Pathology* **45,** 209.
Schlang, H. A. (1961). *Aerospace Medicine* **32,** 333.
Schlenker, F. S., Taylor, N. A. and Kiehn, B. P. (1964). *American Journal of Clinical Pathology* **42,** 349.
Schmid, R., Schwartz, S. and Watson, C. J. (1950). *Proceedings of the Society for Experimental Biology and Medicine* **75,** 705.
Schroeder, H. A. (1960a). *Journal of the American Medical Association* **172,** 1902.
Schroeder, H. A. (1960b). *Journal of Chronic Diseases* **12,** 586.
Schroeder, H. A. (1966). *Journal of the American Medical Association* **195,** 81.
Schroeder, H. A. and Balassa, J. J. (1961). *Journal of Chronic Diseases* **14,** 408.

Schroeder, H. A. and Mitchener, M. (1971). *Archives of Environmental Health* **23,** 102.
Schroeder, H. A. and Tipton, I. H. (1968). *Archives of Environmental Health* **17,** 965.
Schroeder, H. A., Balassa, J. J. and Vinton, W. H. (1964). *Journal of Nutrition* **83,** 239.
Schroeder, H. A., Balassa, J. J. and Vinton, W. H. (1965). *Journal of Nutrition* **86,** 51.
Schroeder, H. A., Vinton, W. H. and Balassa, J. J. (1963a). *Journal of Nutrition* **80,** 39.
Schroeder, H. A., Vinton, W. H. and Balassa, J. J. (1963b). *Journal of Nutrition* **80,** 48.
Schroeder, H. A., Mitchener, M. and Nason, A. P. (1970). *Journal of Nutrition* **100,** 59.
Schroeder, T., Avery, D. D. and Cross, H. A. (1972). *Experientia* **28,** 425.
Schubert, J. and White, M. P. (1952). *Journal of Laboratory and Clinical Medicine* **39,** 260.
Schwartz, K. and Mertz, W. (1959). *Archives of Biochemistry and Biophysics* **85,** 292.
Schwartz, S. (1951). *In* "Toxicity of Uranium" (A. Tannenbaum ed.) p. 290. McGraw-Hill, New York.
Secchi, G. C., Ambrosi, L. and Rezzonico, A. (1968). *Medicina del Lavoro* **59,** 593.
Secchi, G. C., Alessio, L., Cambiaghi, G. and Andreoletti, F. (1972). International Symposium, Environmental Health Aspects of Lead, Amsterdam, Paper, 56.
Selander, S. and Cramér, K. (1970). *British Journal of Industrial Medicine* **27,** 28.
Selander, S., Cramér, K. and Hallberg, L. (1966). *British Journal of Industrial Medicine* **23,** 282.
Selariu, C. and Milhăescu, S. (1957). *Comunicările Academiei Republicii Populare Române* **7,** 45.
Selye, H. and Somogyi, A. (1968). *Archives of Environmental Health* **16,** 827.
Selye, H., Tuchweber, B. and Bertók, L. (1961). *Journal of Bacteriology* **91,** 884.
Selye, H., Caruso, P. L., Tuchweber, B. and Gabbiani, G. (1964a). *Annals of Allergy* **22,** 645.
Selye, H., Gabbiani, G. and Seratimov, N. (1964b). *Journal of Histochemistry and Cytochemistry* **12,** 563.
Selye, H., Gabbiani, G. and Tuchweber, B. (1964c). *Neurology* **14,** 1084.
Seppäläinen, A. M. and Hernberg, S. (1972). *British Journal of Industrial Medicine* **29,** 443.
Sessa, T., Farrari, E. and Colucci, C. (1965). *Folia Medica (Napoli)* **48,** 658.
Sheets, R. F., Janney, C. D., Hamilton, H. E. and De Gowin, E. L. (1951). *Journal of Clinical Investigation* **30,** 1272.
Sherer, J. W. (1935). *Missouri Medicine* **32,** 275.
Shields, J. B. and Mitchell, H. H. (1941). *Journal of Nutrition* **21,** 541.
Shields, J. B., Mitchell, H. H. and Ruth, W. A. (1938). *Journal of Industrial Hygiene* **21,** 7.
Shimazono, J. (1914). *Archives of Psychiatry* **53,** 972.
Shimizu, Y. (1965). *Zeitschrifte für Zellforschung und Mikroskopische Anatomie* **67,** 185.
Shupe, J. L., Binns, W., James, L. F. and Keeler, R. F. (1967). *Journal of the American Veterinary Medical Association* **151,** 198.
Simpson, J. A., Seaton, D. A. and Adams, J. F. (1964). *Journal of Neurology, Neurosurgery and Psychiatry* **27,** 536.
Singer, M. J. and Hanson, L. (1969). *Proceedings of the Soil Science Society of America* **33,** 152.
Singerland, W. (1955). *Journal of Clinical Endocrinology* **15,** 131.
Singerman, A. (1964). *Archives of Environmental Health* **9,** 464.
Sinyakova, S. I. (1945). *Compte Rendu de l'Académie des Sciences de l'U.R.S.S.* **48,** 648.
Six, K. M. and Goyer, R. A. (1970). *Journal of Laboratory and Clinical Medicine* **76,** 933.
Six, K. M. and Goyer, R. A. (1972). *Journal of Laboratory and Clinical Medicine* **79,** 128.
Skaar, H., Ophus, E. and Gullvåg, B. M. (1973). *Nature* **241,** 215.

Skripnichenko, Z. M. (1955). *Oftalmologicheskiĭ Zhurnal* **4,** 231.
Skripnichenko, Z. M. (1964). *Oftalmologicheskiĭ Zhurnal* **19,** 597.
Smith, H. D. (1964). *Archives of Environmental Health* **8,** 256.
Smith, H. D., Baehner, R. L., Carney, T. and Majors, W. J. (1963). *American Journal of Diseases of Children* **105,** 609.
Snyder, L. J. (1967). *Analytical Chemistry* **39,** 591.
Sobel, A. E. and Burger, M. (1955). *Journal of Biological Chemistry* **212,** 105.
Sobel, A. E., Grawon, O. and Kremer, B. (1938). *Proceedings of the Society for Experimental Biology and Medicine* **38,** 433.
Sobel, A. E., Yusaka, H., Peters, D. D. and Kremer, B. (1940). *Journal of Biological Chemistry* **132,** 239.
Soldatović, D. and Petrović, C. (1963). *Archives de Farmacia* **13,** 253.
Soldatović, D., Djurović, M. and Petrović, C. (1966). *Archives de Farmacia* **16,** 151.
Soliman, M., El-Sadek, Y. and El-Waseef, A. (1972). International Symposium, Environmental Health Aspects of Lead, Amsterdam, Paper 49.
Sonkin, N. (1963). *New England Journal of Medicine* **269,** 779.
Sorensen, L. L. C. and Nobe, K. (1972). *Environmental Science and Technology* **6,** 239.
Speizer, F. E., Ferris, B. G., Burgess, W. A. and Kopito, L. K. (1972). International Symposium, Environmental Health Aspects of Lead, Amsterdam, Paper 78.
Srivastava, P. C. and Umadi, S. (1968). *British Medical Journal* **1,** 578.
Sroczyński, J. and Jonderko, G. (1963). *Postepy Higieny i Medycyny Doświadozalnej* **17,** 609.
Sroczyński, J. and Kossmann, S. (1966). *Polish Medical Journal* **5,** 85.
Sroczyński, J. and Kossmann, S. (1967). *Patologia Polska* **18,** 149.
Sroczyński, J. and Pierkarski, B. (1959). *Postepy Higieny i Medycyny Doświadozalnej* **13,** 781.
Sroczyński, J. and Zajusz, K. (1966). *Archivum Immunologiæ et Therapiæ Experimentalis* **14,** 391.
Sroczyński, J., Buczkowski, M. and Wieczorek, M. (1954). *Med. Pracy.* **15,** 139.
Sroczyński, J., Jonderko, G. and Watras, J. (1964). *Proceedings of the 10th Congress of the International Society of Haematology, Stockholm,* p. 184.
Sroczyński, J., Jonderko, G. and Watras, J. (1966). *Arch. Immunol. Ther. exp.* **14,** 536.
Stanford Research Institute (1956). "Literature Review of Metropolitan Air Pollutant Concentrations: Preparation, Sampling and Assay of Synthetic Atmospheres."
Stanković, M. and Mokranjac, M. (1964). *Proceedings of the 14th International Congress on Occupational Health, Madrid,* Vol. 2, p. 831.
Stanković, M., Poleti, D. and Petrović, L. (1960). *Proceedings of the 13th International Congress on Occupational Health, New York,* p. 368.
Stanković, M., Djurić, D., D. Milić, S. and Djordjevic, V. (1972). International Symposium, Environmental Health Aspects of Lead, Amsterdam, Paper 47.
Staples, E. L. J. 1955). *New Zealand Veterinary Journal* **3,** 39.
Sterling, T. D. (1964). *Archives of Environmental Health* **8,** 333.
Sterling, T. D., Kehoe, R. A. and Rustagi, J. S. (1964). *Archives of Environmental Health* **8,** 44.
Stern, A. C. (Ed.) (1968) *In* "Air Pollution" p. 668, 2nd ed., Vol. 3, Academic Press, New York.
Stewart, C. M. (1966). *Science* **153,** 1068.
Stich, W. (1961). *Klinische Wochenschrift* **39,** 338.
Stitt, F. W., Clayton, D. G., Crawford, M. D. and Morris, J. N. (1973). *Lancet* **1,** 122.
Stocken, L. A. and Thompson, R. H. S. (1949). *Physiological Reviews* **29,** 168.

Stöfen, D. (1966). *Zentralblatt für Arbeitsmedizin und Arbeitsschutz* **16,** 11.
Stöfen, D. (1968). *Archiv für Hygiene und Bakteriologie* **52,** 93.
Stöfen, D. (1969a). *Archiv für Hygiene und Bakteriologie* **153,** 380.
Stöfen, D. (1969b). *Zuchthygiene* **4,** 169.
Stöfen, D. (1970). *Städtehygiene* **21,** 94.
Stöfen, D. (1971). *Städtehygiene* **22,** 171.
Stokinger, A. E. and Mountain, J. T. (1967). *Journal of Occupational Medicine* **9,** 537.
Stover, B. J. (1959). *Proceedings of the Society for Experimental Biology and Medicine* **100,** 269.
Strauss, H., Geleriu, R. and Ionut, C. (1972). International Symposium, Environmental Health Aspects of Lead, Amsterdam, Paper 24.
Strong, J. P., Correa, P. and Solberg, L. (1968). *Laboratory Investgation* **18,** 620.
Stubbs, R. L. (1972). *In* "Lead in the Environment" (P. Hepple ed.) p. 1. Institute of Petroleum, London.
Suchodoller, A. (1967). Thesis, Zurich.
Sutherland, D. A. and Eisentraut, A. M. (1956). *Blood* **11,** 1024.
Suzutani, T. and Taira, H. (1962). *Wakayama Medical Reports* **7,** 29.
Szadkowski, D. and Lehnert, G. (1972). International Symposium, Environmental Health Aspects of Lead, Amsterdam, Paper 74.
Tanabe, Y. (1959). *Japanese Journal of the Nation's Heath* **28,** 386.
Tanford, C. (1950). *Journal of the American Chemical Society* **72,** 441.
Tange, J. D., Hayward, N. J. and Bremner, D. A. (1965). *Australasian Annals of Medicine* **14,** 49.
Tanquerel des Planches, L. (1839). "Traité des Maladies de Plomb ou Saturnines." Ferra, Paris.
Tatsumoto, M. and Patterson, C. C. (1963). *Nature* **199,** 350.
Taylor, A. and Carmichael, N. (1953). *Cancer Studies* **2,** 36.
Teisinger, J. (1935). *Biochemische Zeitschrift* **277,** 178.
Teisinger, J. (1964). *Archiv za Higijenu Rada i Toksikolgiju* **15,** 243.
Teisinger, J. (1966). *Folia Medica (Napoli)* **49,** 421.
Teisinger, J. (1971). *Archives of Environmental Health* **23,** 280.
Teisinger, J. and Srbová, J. (1959). *British Journal of Industrial Medicine* **16,** 148.
Teisinger, J., Zumanová, R. and Zezula, I. (1958). *Archives of Industrial Health* **17,** 295.
Telfer, J. G. (1947). *Journal of the American Medical Association* **135,** 835.
Tepper, L. B. (1963). *Archives of Environmental Health* **7,** 82.
Ter Haar, G. (1970). *Environmental Science and Technology* **4,** 226.
Ter Haar, G. and Bayard, M. A. (1971). *Nature* **232,** 553.
Ter Haar, G., Holtzman, R. B. and Lucas, H. F. (1967). *Nature* **216,** 353.
Ter Haar, G., Lenane, D. L., Hu, J. N. and Brandt, M. (1972). *Journal of the Air Pollution Control Association* **22,** 39.
Thoelin, H., Richterich, R., Pletscher, A. and Staub, H. (1952). *Archiv für Experimentelle Pathologie und Pharmakologie* **215,** 389.
Thomas, H. V., Milmore, B. K., Heidbreder, G. A. and Kogan, B. A. (1967). *Archives of Environmental Health* **15,** 695.
Thomas, P. K. and Lascelles, R. G. (1966). *Quarterly Journal of Medicine* **35,** 489.
Thomas, P. K. and Lascelles, R. G. (1967). *Quarterly Journal of Medicine* **36,** 223.
Thompson, J. A. (1971). *British Journal of Industrial Medicine* **28,** 195.
Thurston, D. L., Middlekamp, J. N. and Mason, E. (1955). *Journal of Pediatrics* **47,** 413.
The Times, 7 December 1968.
Tims, J. M. (1971). *Petroleum Review,* **25,** 228.
Tipton, I. H. and Cook, M. J. (1963). *Health Physics* **9,** 103.

Tipton, I. H and Schaefer, J. J. (1964). *Archives of Environmental Health* **8,** 58.
Tipton, I. H., Schroeder, H. A., Perry, H. M. and Cook, M. J. (1965). *Health Physics* **11,** 403.
Tishkoff, G. W., Granville, N. B., Rosen, R. and Damashek, W. (1958). *Acta haematologica* **19,** 321.
Tolan, A. and Elton, G. (1972). International Symposium, Environmental Health Aspects of Lead, Amsterdam, Paper 3.
Tompsett, S. L. (1956). *Analyst* **81,** 330.
Tonomura, M., Nanjo, M. and Kano, S. (1965). *Bulletin of the National Institute of Hygiene Science, Tokyo* **83,** 81.
Totovic, V. (1965). *Virchows Archiv für Pathologische Anatomie und Physiologie und für Klinische Medizin* **339,** 151.
Tredgold, A. F. (1947). "Mental Deficiency", 7th edition. Ballière, Tindall and Cox, London.
de Treville, R. (1964). *Archives of Environmental Health* **8,** 212.
Truffert, L., Lebbe, J. and Chovin, P. (1966). *Zeitschrift für Präventivmedizin* **11,** 134.
Truscott, R. B. (1970). *Canadian Journal of Comparative Medicine and Veterinary Science* **34,** 134.
Tschudy, D. P. (1969). *In* "Duncan's Diseases of Metabolism" (P. K. Bondy and L. E. Rosenberg eds.) 6th edition, p. 600. W. B. Saunders, Philadelphia.
Tschudy, D. P., Perlroth, M. G., Marver, H. S., Collins, A., Hunter, G. and Rechcigl, M. (1965). *Proceedings of the National Academy of Sciences of the U.S.A.* **53,** 841.
Tsuchiya, K. (1964). *Industrial Health* **2,** 162.
Tuttle, A. H. and Fitch, C. (1958). *American Journal of Diseases of Children* **96,** 503.
Tylecote, R. F. (1964). *British Journal of the History of Science* **2,** 25.
United States Department of Health, Education and Welfare (1965). "Survey of Lead in the Atmosphere of Three Urban Communities." Public Health Service Publication No. 999-AP-12.
United States Environmental Protection Agency (1972). "Health Hazards of Lead, Report of the U.S. E.P.A.'s Bureau of Air Pollution Sciences." Washington.
Urbanowicz, H. (1971). *Archives of Environmental Health* **23,** 284.
Van Assen, F. J. J. (1958). *Nederlands Tijdschrift voor verloskunde en Gynecologie* **58,** 258.
Vannotti, A. and Imholz, A. (1939). *Zeitschrift für die Gesamte Experimentelle Medizin* **106,** 597.
Vardanis, A. and Quastel, J. H. (1961). *Canadian Journal of Biochemistry* **39,** 1811.
Verloop, M. C., Bierenga, M. and Diezeraad-Njoo, A. (1962). *Acta haematologica* **27,** 129.
Vial, J. D. (1958). *Journal of Biophysical and Biochemical Cytology* **4,** 551.
Vigdorchik, N. A. (1935). *Journal of Industrial Hygiene* **17,** 1.
Vigliani, E. C. (1950). *Medicina del Deporte y del Trabajo* **85,** 3118.
Vigliani, E. C. and Angeleri, C. (1935). *Clinica Medica Italiana* **66,** 5.
de Villaverde, J. M. (1929–1930). *Trabajos del Instituto Cajal de Investigaciones Biológicas* **26,** 163.
Vincent, P. C. (1958). *Australian Journal of Experimental Biology and Medical Science* **36,** 589.
Vinogradov, A. P. (1946). *Chemical Abstracts* **40,** 1892.
Vinogradov, A. P. (1954). "Geochemie Seltener und nur in Spuren Vorhandener Chemischer Elemente in Boden." Akademische Verlagsgesellschaft Berlin.
Vitale, L. F., Fine, B. P., Barth, A. and Filkin, K. (1972). *Pediatrics* **81,** 977.
Vogt, E. C. (1930). *American Journal of Roentgenology* **24,** 550.

Vogt, E. C. (1932). *Journal of the American Medical Association* **98,** 125.

Volhard, F. and Fahr, T. (1914). "Die Brightsche Nierenkrankheit." Springer, Berlin.

Vostál, J. (1963). *Biochemical Pharmacology* **12,** Suppl. 207.

Vostál, J. (1966). *Proceedings of the 15th International Congress on Occupational Health, Vienna*, Vol. 3, p. 61.

Vostál, J. and Heller, J. (1968). *Environmental Research* **2,** 1.

Wachstein, M. (1949). *Archives of Pathology* **48,** 442.

Waggener, J. D., Bunn, S. M. and Beggs, J. (1965). *Journal of Neuropathology and Experimental Neurology* **24,** 430.

Waksman, B. H., Adams, R. D. and Mansmann, H. L. (1957). *Journal of Experimental Medicine* **105,** 591.

Waldman, R. K. and Borman, E. K. (1959). *Archives of Industrial Health* **19,** 431.

Waldron, H. A. (1964a). *British Journal of Industrial Medicine* **21,** 315.

Waldron, H. A. (1964b). *Journal of Clincal Pathology* **17,** 149.

Waldron, H. A. (1964c). *Journal of Clinical Pathology* **17,** 405.

Waldron, H. A. (1965). *Journal of Clinical Pathology* **18,** 230.

Waldron, H. A. (1966). *British Journal of Industrial Medicine* **23,** 83.

Waldron, H. A. (1971). *British Journal of Industrial Medicine* **28,** 195.

Waller, R. E., Commins, B. T. and Lawther, P. J. (1965). *British Journal of Industrial Medicine* **22,** 128.

Walshe, J. M. (1956). *American Journal of Medicine* **21,** 487.

Warley, F. W., Blackledge, P. and O'Gorman, P. (1968). *British Medical Journal* **1,** 117.

Warren, H. V. (1959). *Nature* **184,** 561.

Warren, H. V. (1961). *Canadian Journal of Public Health* **52,** 157.

Warren, H. V. (1963). *Practitioner* **6,** 517.

Warren, H. V. and Delavault, R. E. (1960). *Transactions of the Royal Society of Canada, Section III* **54,** 11.

Warren, H. V. and Delavault, R. E. (1962). *Journal of the Science of Food and Agriculture* **13,** 96.

Warren, H. V., Delavault, R. E. and Cross, C. H. (1967). *Annals of the New York Academy of Science* **136,** 657.

Warren, H. V., Delavault, R. E., Fletcher, K. and Wilks, E. (1971). *Western Miner (February)*.

Watanabe, G. and Yana, T. (1953). *Archives of Industrial Hygiene* **7,** 444.

Watson, C. J. (1950). *Archives of Internal Medicine* **86,** 797.

Watson, C. J., Hawkinson, V. and Bossenmaier, I. (1953). *Transactions of the Association of American Physicians* **66,** 144.

Watson, R. J., Decker, E. and Lichtman, H. (1958). *Pediatrics* **21,** 40.

Waxman, H. S. and Rabinowitz, M. (1966). *Biochimica et Biophysica Acta* **129,** 369.

Weatherall, M. (1948). *British Journal of Pharmacology* **3,** 137.

Weatherall, M. (1954). *Pharmacological Reviews* **6,** 133.

Webster, H. de F., Spiro, D., Waksman, B. B. and Adams, R. N. (1961). *Journal of Neuropathology and Experimental Neurology* **20,** 5.

Webster, H. de F., Schroeder, J. M., Asbury, A. K. and Adams, R. D. (1967). *Journal of Neuropathology and Experimental Neurology* **26,** 276.

Wechsler, W. and Hager, H. (1962). *Beiträge zur Pathologischen Anatomie und zur Allgemeinen Pathologie* **126,** 252.

Weiner, G. (1970). *Public Health Reports* **85,** 19.

Weinig, E. and Börner, B. (1961). *Archiv für Toxikologie* **19,** 34.

Weir, P. A. and Hine, C. H. (1970). *Archives of Environmental Health* **20,** 45.

Weiss, D. (1972). Thesis, Michigan Technological University.
Weiss, D., Whitten, B. and Leddy, D. (1972). *Science* **178,** 69.
Weissberg, J. B., Lipschutz, F. and Oski, F. A. (1971). *New England Journal of Medicine* **284,** 565.
Weller, R. O. (1965). *Journal of Pathology and Bacteriology* **89,** 591.
Weller, R. O. (1967). *Journal of Neurology, Neurosurgery and Psychiatry* **30,** 111.
Westerman, M. P. and Jensen, W. N. (1963). *Journal of Clinical Investigation* **42,** 991.
Westerman, M. P., Pfitzer, E., Ellis, L. D. and Jensen, W. N. (1965). *New England Journal of Medicine* **273,** 1246.
Whitaker, J. A. and Vietti, T. J. (1958). *Pediatrics* **24,** 734.
Whitaker, J. A., Austin, W. and Nelson, J. D. (1962). *Pediatrics* **29,** 384.
White, H. H. and Fowler, F. D. (1960). *Pediatrics,* **25,** 309.
Whitehead, T. P. and Prior, A.P. (1960). *Lancet* **2,** 1343.
Whitfield, C. L., Ch'ien, L. T. and Whitehead, J. D. (1972). *American Journal of Medicine* **53,** 289.
Wiklander, L. (1970). *Grundoerbattring* **23,** 163.
Williams, C. (1911). *Annals of Ophthalmology* **20,** 719.
Williams, H. W., Caraway, W. T. and de Young, W. A. (1954). *Archives of Neurology and Psychiatry* **72,** 579.
Williams, J. D., Leigh, D. A. and Matthews, G. A. (1966). *Annals of Occupational Hygiene* **9,** 1.
Williams, M. K. (1965). Thesis, Oxford.
Williams, M. K. (1966). *British Journal of Industrial Medicine* **23,** 105.
Williams, M. K. (1971). *New Scientist* **49,** 578.
Williams, M. K. (1972). *Lancet* **2,** 480.
Williams, M. K., King, E. and Walford, J. (1968), *British Medical Journal* **1,** 618.
Williams, M. K., King, E. and Walford, J. (1969). *British Journal of Industrial Medicine* **26,** 202.
Wilson, A. T. (1965). M.D. Thesis, Edinburgh.
Wilson, A. T. (1967). *Lancet* **1,** 956.
Wilson, S. A. K. (1907). *Review of Neurology and Psychiatry* **5,** 441.
Wilson, V. K., Thomson, M. L. and Dent, C. E. (1953). *Lancet* **2,** 66.
Winchester, J. W., Zoller, W. H., Duce, R. A. and Benson, C. S. (1967). *Atmospheric Environment* **1,** 105.
Windeyer Committee (1972). "Report of a Committee under the Chairmanship of Sir Brian Windeyer Appointed to Inquire into Lead Poisoning at the RTZ Smelter at Avonmouth." H.M.S.O., London.
Withers, S. (1930). *American Journal of Roentology* **24,** 169.
Witschi, H. P. (1964). *Archiv für Gewerbepathologie und Gewerbehygiene* **20,** 449.
Wittgens, H. and Niederstadt, D. (1954). *Zentralblatt für Arbeitsmedizin und Arbeitsschutz* **4,** 185.
Wittgens, H. and Niederstadt, D. (1955). *Archiv für Gewerbepathologie und Gewerbehygiene* **13,** 544.
Wolman, M. (1954). *Journal of Pathology and Bacteriology* **68,** 159.
Woods, G. E. and Walters, R. M. (1964). *Lancet* **2,** 592.
World Health Organization (1970). "European Standards for Drinking Water." W.H.O., Geneva.
World Health Organization (1971). "International Standards for Drinking Water." W.H.O., Geneva.

Wright, J. R., Levick, R. and Atkinson, H. J. (1955). *Proceedings of the Soil Science Society of America* **19,** 340.

Wyllie, J. (1955). *Archives of Industrial Health* **12,** 396.

Wynne, F. E. (1911). *British Medical Journal* **2,** 267.

Yagihara, T. (1960). *Annales Paediatrici Japonici* **6,** 489.

Yaverbaum, P. M. (1963). *Gigiena Truda i Professīonal'nȳe zaldevanīya* **7,** 38.

Zahorski, W. and Myślak, Z. (1957). *Proceedings of the 12th International Congress on Occupational Health, Helsinki,* Vol. 3, p. 242.

Zegarski, W. (1963). *Acta Biologica et Medica Societas Scientiarum Gedanensis* **7,** 33.

Ziegfield, R. L. (1964). *Archives of Environmental Health* **8,** 202.

Zielhuis, R. L. (1971). *Archives of Environmental Health* **23,** 299.

Zollinger, H. U. (1953). *Virchows Archiv für Pathologische Anatomie und Physiologie und für Klinische Medizine* **323,** 694.

Zook, B. C., Carpenter, J. L. and Leeds, E. B. (1969). *Journal of the American Veterinary Medical Association* **155,** 1329.

Zook, B. C., Sauer, R. M. and Garner, F. M. (1970). *Journal of the American Veterinary Medical Association* **157,** 691.

Zuliani, G. Perin, G. and Rausa, G. (1966). *Medicina del Lavoro* **57,** 771.

Author Index

Numbers in *italics* indicate pages where references are listed in full.

C

D

E

F

I

J

R

S

Subject Index